stuttering therapy:

prevention and intervention with children

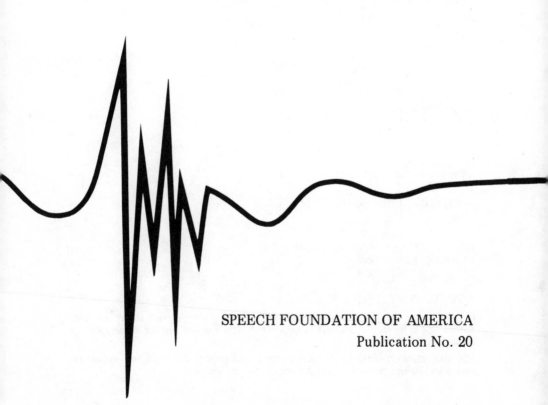

SPEECH FOUNDATION OF AMERICA

Publication No. 20

1st PRINTING—1985
2nd PRINTING—1986

Speech Foundation of America
P. O. Box 11749
Memphis, Tennessee 38111

Library of Congress Number 86-051054
ISBN 0-933388-22-5

The Speech Foundation of America is a non-profit charitable organization dedicated to the prevention and therapy of stuttering.

Contents

preface 7
    Jane Fraser

chapter one
    Emotional and Environmental Problems
    In Stuttering 9
    Dean E. Williams, Ph.D.

chapter two
    Language Formulation Related
    To Disfluency and Stuttering 19
    Lois A. Nelson, Ph.D.

chapter three
    Speech Motor Processes and Stuttering in Children;
    A Theoretical and Clinical Perspective 39
    John M. Hanley, Ph.D.

chapter four
    The Development of Fluency in Normal Children 67
    C. Woodruff Starkweather, Ph.D.

chapter five
    Toward a Therapy Assessment Procedure
    For Treating Stuttering in Children 101
    Roger J. Ingham, Ph.D.

chapter six
    Integration: Present Status and Prospects
    For the Future 130
    Hugo H. Gregory, Ph.D.

Preface

Almost every conference and resulting publication of the Speech Foundation of America has focused, in one way or another, on improving intervention with children who stutter. Today, there is general agreement among clinicians that considerable progress has been made in understanding the gradations of difference between normal disfluency and stuttering, in evaluating children showing varying degrees of stuttering, and in carrying out effective therapy. Most important of all, appropriate counseling of parents and therapeutic interaction with children is leading in many cases to the prevention of stuttering after rather short-term intervention of four to eight weeks.

The 1982 conference, "Evaluation of Disfluency, Prevention of Stuttering, and Management of Fluency Problems in Children", at Northwestern University was one in which 105 professional clinicians from speech-language pathology, psychology, and psychiatry came together to hear five presentations about developmental and environmental factors related to the onset of stuttering, evaluation and treatment procedures, and the measurement of therapy outcome. Following each presentation, subgroups of participants discussed each paper and posed questions that were then presented to the speakers for additional comment. In this way, the experiences of participants from the United States, Canada, Europe, and Central America were shared. Lively conversation about conference topics continued during meals together and as small groups gathered between sessions.

It is not possible to measure the impact of such a conference, but many have written to us or told various participants of the way in which the content of this meeting has influenced their subsequent work. To share in yet another way and to continue the process of developing and consolidating ideas, the six papers given at the conference are being made available in this publication. The last of these papers is an integration of the main points made in individual papers and in discussion groups.

Members of the conference planning committee were the following:

Hugo H. Gregory, Ph.D., Northwestern University
Barry Guitar, Ph.D., University of Vermont
Harold Luper, Ph.D., University of Tennessee
Theodore Peters, Ph.D., University of Wisconsin
C. Woodruff Starkweather, Ph.D., Temple University
Dean Williams, Ph.D., University of Iowa

We are grateful to these authorities for their time and for their ideas about how topics should be covered. (Jane Fraser represented the Speech Foundation of America in planning the conference.)

Harold Luper, Ph.D., served as conference coordinator. It was fortunate to have Dr. Luper handle this task and to have the following other prominent contributors serve as discussion leaders:

> Martin Adams, Ph.D., University of Houston
> Einer Boberg, Ph.D., University of Alberta
> Edward Conture, Ph.D., Syracuse University
> Barry Guitar, Ph.D., University of Vermont
> Theodore Peters, Ph.D., University of Wisconsin
> Glydon Riley, Ph.D., California State University
> Lena Rustin, British Health Authority
> Frank Stournaras
> Academic Hospital, Erasmus University, Holland

Yolande Mallian served as Conference Secretary. In this role she worked many hours to make arrangements and handle correspondence.

The five presenters at the conference worked diligently before and after the conference with the editor of this publication, Hugo H. Gregory, Ph.D., to provide a contemporary analysis of their topics including the delineation of specific techniques that can be used in the evaluation and treatment of children who stutter. They join with the planning committee and with us in hoping that you will find this information useful in your clinical work.

> Jane Fraser
> President, Speech Foundation of America

chapter one

Emotional and Environmental Problems in Stuttering

Dean E. Williams, Ph.D.
University of Iowa

Before we can discuss meaningful things clinicians can do to prevent stuttering or to manage fluency problems, we must establish some foundation for what it is we are attempting to prevent or to manage.

Researchers are still as far from distinguishing between a "beginning stutter," and a normal disfluency as they were forty years ago. This fact should not be forgotten. The problem will not go away by pretending it does not exist—or by exclaiming "we all know what we mean." We do not. For clinical purposes, and for the purposes of this conference, ordinarily—not always—but usually—we can agree when a child is showing "signs" of a fluency problem. Research data (Johnson, 1959) (VanRiper, 1982) indicate that it usually begins, but not always, between two and one-half and four years of age. Usually, but not always, the child talks normally for one to two years before a problem begins. Easy repetitions with no accompanying tension or laryngeal "blockings" are usually, but not always, the first behavior evaluated as "trouble." Usually, but not always, the problem develops gradually not suddenly. Parents report on the average that it was approximately five to six months between the time when they first noticed the child do "something" and the time they decided that there was a fluency problem.

The above summary of current knowledge should serve to keep us humble, questioning, and open minded. Certainly, it should negate the influence of anyone who attempts to purport a single, simple answer to complex problems.

VanRiper (1982) was certainly aware of the complexity of identifying stuttering when he presented twenty six behaviors as guidelines to assist the clinician differentiate between stuttering and normal disfluency in children. These guidelines focus on two main aspects of the child's behavior. The first differentiates the nature, type, frequency and duration of the speech disfluencies. The second reflect behavioral indications of reactions of the child to the ways he is talking. We must keep the major point in front of us, however, that these are just guidelines—not absolutes. The most valid conclusion that can be drawn is that *the more* of the differentiating behaviors that the child demonstrates, the *more likely* it is that he is developing or will develop a problem of clinical significance.

At the time that most stuttering develops (3-4 years of age) the child is undergoing a neuromotor, cognitive, and emotional spurt in growth. Many children experience a relative increase in disfluencies at this time. For most, the increase is temporary. For some few, the increase is quite marked and persistent. These few are the ones who are likely to develop stuttering. Therefore, we are faced on the one hand with the need to understand why certain children are more disfluent than others and, on the other hand, to develop efficient procedures for reducing a child's frequency and duration of disfluencies.

Current researchers on stuttering are, for the most part, focusing their interest on the *person* who stutters. Earlier in this conference in her chapter Nelson has discussed the expressive and receptive language abilities of stutterers. Results from studies differ but there seems to be little doubt that some children who have differences in language development exhibit increased disfluencies and stuttering. In another chapter Hanley discussed research findings on the speed and timing of the motor responses of stutterers. With some adult stutterers, at least, there appear to be deficiencies in this area. We must await future research in order to further delineate the range and extent of such deficiencies. After that, researchers must determine how a certain deficiency may—or may not—result in stuttering. Therefore, continued investigation of the speech and language production abilities of the child who stutters is of vital importance.

Not too many years ago, the emphasis in research was on determining those conditions in the child's environment that increased disfluencies in speech. The focus here was not so much on speech production abilities but on disturbed communication. As such, it included a study of those interactions between speaker and listener that are the important elements in communication. Research interest in this area has diminished in recent years. This, to me, is unfortunate because I believe that in a few years it will become obvious that stuttering develops as a result of an interaction between the child's abilities, and disturbed communication. Conture (1982) states it clearly:

> Stuttering most likely results from a complex interaction between the stutterer's environment—and the abilities the stutterer brings to that environment. (p. 18)

Conture emphasizes the interaction *between* environment and individual abilities. Let us now examine those factors *within* the environment—emotional, cognitive, verbal and nonverbal stresses in *personal interactions*—that can disturb a child's developing verbal communication abilities. One of the ways this can be evidenced is by increased disfluency.

Emotional Factors in Stuttering

Before we consider emotional conditions within the child's environment that can increase speech disfluencies, we should review the information available about the emotional stability of the child who begins to stutter and of his parents.

For years the adult stutterer has undergone extensive examination under the psychological testing microscope. There have been far too many studies for one to review them here. Bloodstein (1975), after reviewing the major studies concluded that most stutterers perform well within the norms. Most certainly the results preclude a conclusion of their being a definable stuttering personality. Generally, as Sheehan (1970) reported, adult stutterers show rather consistently lower levels of aspiration and higher levels of anxiety in situations involving speech. Children who stutter show no definable personality differences from normal speaking children. The fact that adult stutterers as a group are not quite as well adjusted as nonstuttering adults, to me, is not surprising. If they were, I would conclude that they either were neurotic, or insensitive, or just not aware of what is going on around them.

The parents of stutterers also have received considerable

attention. Again, as with the stutterers, it is beyond the scope of this paper to review them here. Bloodstein (1975) has reviewed the research and summarized the findings. Johnson (1959) and his students have found that many parents of stutterers when compared to parents of nonstutterers generally and in different specific ways put more pressure on their child to perform according to their relatively high standards. These findings have been corroborated by independent research. Andrews and Harris (1964), on the other hand, studying mothers of stutterers in England found them to be of low innate capacity and creating an unstable home environment. Also, the stutterers showed late and poor speech development. As Bloodstein mentions, both the Johnson and the Andrews and Harris studies may point to reasons for the development of stuttering. I emphasize it here for the implications that result from the ways we historically have thought about stuttering. For too long we have thought of it as a unitary phenomenon that results from a single cause and evolves into a homogeneous entity. That, for example, is why most of our research concerned with the emotional stability of the stutterer has attempted to find definitive differences between stutterers and nonstutterers as a group. Yet, clinically, most of us have observed *individual* children who have shown extreme emotional reactions to environmental pressures that resulted in a dramatic increase in disfluencies. Most of these, according to my experiences, have evolved in conjunction with family problems. In fact, any time I find a child whose disfluencies—usually part or whole word repetitions and/or prolongations often accompanied by obvious emotional distress, i.e., tensing, struggling, crying, yelling, etc.—began suddenly and with high frequency, I look for factors in the home that could account for such reactions by the child. These conditions have included, in my experience, such things as: (1) birth of a sibling where the child's status and way of life is shattered; (2) relatively extreme changes in disciplinary practices; (3) going to preschool when, at the same time, hearing their parents talk about how great it is to have them gone from home for a time; (4) verbal bickering, fighting, or separation by the parents; and (5) older sibling(s) who torment, dictate, talk for and/or tease the child. These represent only a few examples but they should be sufficient to illustrate the types of family situations to which certain children react through their speech behavior. There is one other fluency problem that I categorize as an "emotional reaction." This is a situation where there is a relatively rapid onset of easy, effortless part or whole word repetitions, high in frequency, and relatively consistent in all speaking situations. The conditions to which the child is reacting are usually more subtle than the ones I mentioned above. They usually involve the loss of individuality in a general sense. They include situations where the child appears to be "lost in the shuffle" of the family's activities. To him, no one pays much attention to what he says or does. There are very few smiles directed to him. There are no pats on the back. No one talks to him much about what he did, plans to do, how he felt, is feeling, or expects to feel. Furthermore, often there are few disciplinary guidelines for him. He gives the impression that little is expected of him.

Generally then, conditions that exist for a child which, *for him*, create considerable inner confusion, sadness, tenseness, anxiety, etc., can result in a disintegration of fluency.

Environmental Factors in Stuttering

For the majority of children who are beginning to stutter, there are not the dramatic emotional problems discussed above. When there is a relative increase in the frequency and/or duration of disfluency for most children, we look for conditions in the environment that are conducive to producing more stress or conflict, for the child. While doing this, we are very much aware that there are certain speaking conditions that result in most speakers being more disfluent than is usually the case. This is true for most adults but it is especially true for children of three or four who are trying to cope with the problems of joining the talking world. In chapter two, Nelson discusses such types of speaking situations. There are other such lists in the literature, for example, VanRiper (1973) and Williams (1978). There is considerable overlap between lists. There are also certain speaking conditions mentioned by one and not by others. This is to be expected. Each clinician constructs the list from his/her own background of experience. The important point for our purposes is that there is a commonality in all of them.

A child will be more disfluent in a *communicative interaction* where he has difficulty coping constructively with the *relative complexity* of the interactions in the face of certain limitations of his own abilities, e.g., neuro-motor integration, language abilities, emotional stability, personal adjustment, etc. Problems of coping with the relative complexity of an interaction can best be understood if we consider first what is meant by good verbal communication. Stated concisely, it involves one person *reaching toward* another with words and the other person reaching *back* with or without words—touching softly. A child is just beginning to learn that one can hit with words, can hurt with words, can kiss with words or can caress with them. Also, the child is just beginning to learn the awesome power of words. Through their use, he can direct the behavior of others and in turn be directed by them. Hopefully, in the midst of all of this, the child will learn the beauty of words by experiencing warm verbal-sharing relationships. Such experiences encourage the child to reach *toward* people in increasingly positive ways resulting in increased speech fluency. At any time disruptive factors invade and sever the invisible threads of the communicative bond between speaker and listener, the child, if he is to speak does so in the presence of a disturbed interaction. Hence, when a relative increase in disfluencies accompany such an interaction, the clinician must deal *not* so much with a *speech problem*, as she must with a *communication problem.*

Verbal communication is affected by the speaker, the listener, and the conditions present as they speak to each other. When a child is beginning to stutter, we usually examine the possible effect of each of those factors in producing stress for the child as he speaks.

First, we look for situations where the stress is self imposed by the child's/speaker's own behaviors. These may include, for example, the times he "talks over his head," his attempted use of vocabulary and sentences too advanced for his abilities, the frequency with which he interrupts other speakers or speaks in competition with others, etc. Next, we look for situations where the stress is imposed by the listener(s), e.g., parents, siblings or friends. These include such times when the listeners do not listen, they interrupt, they finish words or sentences, they hurry the child when he talks. These are only a few examples.

Finally, we explore those conditions present during verbal interactions that may exert undue stress on the child. These may be extremely varied and at times difficult to determine. Usually, they involve a conflict for the child. For example, a child who keeps talking when being admonished to "keep quiet." Or, a child who tries to talk in the middle of parental bickering. Or a child who talks when there are feared consequences for what he says. For example, confessing a wrong doing, or, fear of rejection or ridicule. Or, a child who becomes fearful that the way he talks will be unacceptable. All of these types of conditions produce an ambivalence on the part of the child as to whether he should or should not speak. Such ambivalence can be a powerful fluency disruptor (Sheehan, 1970).

The previous discussion represents a brief overview of the structure a clinician may adopt in exploring those environmental factors that can contribute to a relative—and, at times, a dramatic—increase in speech disfluencies. The focus of the exploration is on disruptors in verbal interaction. Before I move onto a discussion of ways a clinician may assist a child, I want to mention one more parent-child relationship which can exist that may contribute to fluency problems for the child.

Some parents feel tremendous pressure as they shoulder their responsibilities as "parents." They find parenting to be a grim and tiring undertaking. They are "dedicated" to the point of having little fun with their child or with each other. They are likely to place unrealistically high goals and standards for their child. They want perfectionism. They want—and expect—perfectionism not only in their child but also in themselves as parents. This kind of environment makes it difficult for the child to accept calmly and constructively the making of mistakes that is a fundamental part of normal learning.

Most certainly there are emotional and environmental factors that can affect fluency other than the ones I have discussed. One can never be complete because each interaction between two people is unique. My previous discussion should be sufficiently complete to permit us to consider different avenues for remediation of a fluency problem.

Methods of Early Intervention

Ten to twenty years ago the recommendations most often made for early intervention for fluency problems involved modifications in the ways the child was handled in the home. In more recent years there have been approaches used which include direct work with the child and his speech fluency. Costello (1980) for example, describes a program in which she reinforces fluency. Shine (1980) on the other hand works to shape a child's speech into fluency by "easy onset" and "rate control." Obviously, then, clinicians have had success resolving a stuttering problem both by working to modify the child's environment and by working with the child and his speaking behavior. Yet, there are those people who will argue that one way is *the* "correct" way and those who will argue that the other way is *the* "correct" way. Let us not get lost in "either-or" thinking. We know that different factors are related to increased disfluency. It seems reasonable to assume that either of the general approaches to remediation may be more effective with certain children than it will with others. Increased knowledge in this area must await further study.

My purpose in this chapter is limited to discussing ways that a clinician may intervene in a child's interactions with others in his environment that (1) will reduce the frequency and duration of speech disfluencies and/or (2) increase fluency. To do this, a clinician must discuss with the parents their daily routines, their disciplinary practices, their expectations for their child and, generally, their interactions with him. From this information the clinician considers factors that may disrupt the development of warm, positive verbal communication. When such factors emerge, the clinician counsels the parents of ways they can change their behavior so as to promote a more positive verbal interaction. For example, if one or both of the parents interrupts the child frequently as he talks, they are encouraged to not interrupt and to give the child adequate time to express his wants and ideas. Mostly a clinician explores with the parents those speaking situations in which the child is most disfluent and those where he is most fluent. From these, often a picture forms of those interactions that disrupt and those that enhance fluency for the child. This information helps focus the nature of the counseling that follows.

In instances where emotional factors appear to have resulted in fluency failure, parents often need only to understand what they can do to help and they will do it. Frequently, only two or three counseling sessions is all that is required to bring about complete remission of stuttering. The same is often true where the parents feel under pressure to do a "good job" parenting and, as a result, place undue pressure on the child. The very act of discussing their worries, concerns, anxieties and fears with an understanding person serves to clarify their perspective of the ways they are treating the child and of the ways they can change. Again, two to four sessions is often enough.

The situations described above are similar to those discussed by VanRiper (1970) about which he states:

> The person unfamiliar with beginning stuttering might view these remarks about a sudden remission (of stuttering) with some skepticism. We do not. We have repeatedly witnessed the dramatic cessation of stuttering and disfluent behavior in these children. (p. 392)

Most certainly I am not reluctant to discuss with the child the ways he talks and to work to improve fluency directly if that approach appears to be indicated. To me it is not indicated when several counseling sessions with the parents result in increased fluency. Furthermore, as long as emotional factors are operating or high pressure is being brought to bear on the child, direct fluency shaping would be contraindicated. The same conclusions would hold when interviews with the parents indicated that "stuttering" occurred primarily during certain verbal interactions, e.g., at the dinner table or when excited. In this situation, one works with the parents to change the conditions under which the child is speaking. In most instances, my personal preference is to first determine if modifying the nature of the child's interactions results in fluency before I work directly with the child to improve his fluency. If normal speech can be reestablished this way it is, to me, preferable. It is easy to do, takes little time, and the results are stable. Obviously there are clinicians who prefer to proceed in other ways. The important point to be made is that the "I prefer" philosophy reflects to a large extent our state of current knowledge.

We, as clinical scientists, have much work to do in order to determine the most effective means of remediating a beginning fluency problem. In order to do this, we must first develop means of determining the major factors that are contributing to a child's increased disfluency. The major thrust of one's remediation program will be to reduce or to eliminate the influence of those disrupting factors. Fortunately there are those who are beginning to develop structures for differential diagnosis of fluency problems.

Riley and Riley (1979) have developed a component model for diagnosing and treating children who stutter. They separate the factors contributing to increased disfluency into conditions within the child (intrapersonal) and into those outside the child (interpersonal). The intrapersonal factors generally include those associated with language problems plus ones they call "oral motor disorders." The interpersonal factors include those usually associated with disturbed verbal communication. They involve the child and his listeners.

In an article entitled "Stuttering Therapy for Children," Gregory and Hill (1980) describe differential diagnosis procedures that include an indepth evaluation of speech abilities, of language performance and of parent-child interaction. From this they develop a retraining program based on the specific abilities and interactions of the child.

The two reports discussed above reflect, to me, a healthy trend in our profession. We are beginning to investigate those factors within the child and those outside the child that can contribute to increased disfluency. It is from the increased disfluency that a stuttering problem develops. Our focus is shifting from being obsessed with studying a stuttering entity to that of observing and studying a child and his place in the little world in which he lives. From doing this, we can better understand those conditions that—*for him*—influence his speaking performance.

References

Andrews, G., and Harris, M., *The Syndrome of Stuttering*. Clinics in Developmental Med., No. 17. London: Spastics Society Medical Education and Information Unit in association with William Heinemann Medical Books, 1964.

Bloodstein, O., *A Handbook on Stuttering*. Chicago: National Easter Seal Society for Crippled Children and Adults, 1975.

Conture, E. G., *Stuttering*. Englewood Cliffs, New Jersey: Prentice-Hall, 1982.

Costello, J. M., "Operant Conditioning and the Treatment of Stuttering," *Seminars in Speech, Language and Hearing*, Volume 1, Number 4. New York: Thieme-Stratton, Inc., 1980.

Gregory, H. H., and Hill, D., "Stuttering Therapy for Children," *Seminars in Speech, Language and Hearing*, Volume 1, Number 4. New York: Thieme-Stratton, Inc., 1980.

Johnson, W., and Associates, *The Onset of Stuttering*. Minneapolis: University of Minnesota Press, 1959.

Riley, G. D., and Riley, J., "A Component Model for Diagnosing and Treating Children Who Stutter," *Journal of Fluency Disorders*, 4, 279-293, 1979.

Sheehan, J. G., *Stuttering: Research and Therapy*. New York: Harper and Row, 1970.

Shine, R. E., "Direct Management of the Beginning Stutterer," *Seminars in Speech, Language and Hearing*, Volume 1, Number 4. New York: Thieme-Stratton, Inc., 1980.

VanRiper, C., *The Nature of Stuttering, Second Edition*. Englewood Cliffs, New Jersey: Prentice-Hall, 1982.

VanRiper, C., *The Treatment of Stuttering*. Englewood Cliffs, New Jersey: Prentice-Hall, 1973.

Williams, D. E., "Stuttering," *Processes and Disorders of Human Communication*, Curtis, James F. (Ed.). New York: Harper & Row, 1978.

chapter two

Language Formulation Related to Disfluency and Stuttering

Lois A. Nelson, Ph.D.
University of Wisconsin — Madison

There has been an increase in research and clinical observation focusing on the relationships between language developmental factors and disfluency and also language problems in stuttering children. In this chapter, these two areas of study will be reviewed, followed by a discussion of early intervention procedures that include a focus on language factors.

Language Factors and Disfluency

In 1978, Haynes and Hood studied kindergarten children's ability to produce a sentence describing pictures. The examiner had previously modelled grammatically simple and complex sentences for those same pictures. The children were more disfluent when they produced sentences containing complex grammatical constructions.

Pearl and Bernthal (1980) explored the relationship between language usage, as measured on a 30 sentence imitation task, and the occurrence of disfluencies in 30 nonstuttering preschool children. Grammatical complexity of language was controlled through sentences carefully designed to represent 6 different grammatical constructions. When grammatical complexity is controlled, its relationship to disfluency is complicated. Significantly more disfluencies occurred on the passive construction than on the other five types which researchers interpreted as supporting a disfluency/grammatical complexity hypothesis. However, a statistically nonsignificant but high number of disfluencies occurred on the negative construction where few disfluencies were expected. Pearl and Bernthal suggest that semantic complexity (see Slobin 1966) may explain the large number of disfluencies on imitating negative sentences in this study. The five most fluent subjects exhibited 69% of their disfluencies on the sentences that they imitated correctly. The five most disfluent subjects exhibited 80% of their disfluencies on the sentences that they imitated incorrectly and for them the grammatical complexity/disfluency hypothesis was valid. Seventy-six percent of the disfluencies in disfluent subjects occurred at or within one word of the sentence imitation error. This finding suggested to Pearl and Bernthal that some disfluencies were related to sentence processing or to decision points in language formulation. However, the difficulty in imitation tasks is not controlled simply by grammatical complexity. Some researchers argue that we do not know yet what the relationship is between a sentence imitation task and the child's grammatical ability.

Language and Disfluency in Stutterers

Our attention is directed now to young children who are regarded as stutterers. Bloodstein (1974) studied the stuttering of six children and reported that fragmentation occurred at several levels: *word repetition* level which he defined as a fragmenting of a larger element of speech—the phrase, clause or sentence; and *sound and syllable repetition* level which he defined as fragmentation either of the word or of the larger element. For several children every repeated word in the speech sample "is the initial fragment of a sentence, clause, noun phrase, or verb phrase." (1974, p. 389). Only one of Bloodstein's six subjects appeared to fragment words. The others fragmented sentences, clauses, noun phrases, verb phrases, and prepositional phrases. The fragments themselves were primarily word repetitions, although repetitions of sounds, syllables, phrases, and incomplete parts of phrases did occur. He conjectured that for both normal and stuttering children, the repetition of words represents the same kind of fragmentation seen in sound repetition of initial words. It is only that the element of speech is larger.

Bloodstein raised the issue that in its earliest stage, stuttering might be viewed as some type of difficulty in executing whole utterances or the phrase structure within whole utterances. The major influences on the children's stuttering might be the result of "attributes of syntactic structures that cause their motor planning to be more difficult or laborious." (1974, p. 390). Clinically, he speculates that in *early* stuttering, the young child's hesitation in initiating an entire syntactic unit might occur as whole-word repetition. In contrast, the young child who has difficulty initiating words, might exhibit part-word repetition or prolongation. Bloodstein views the latter child as being at a later phase of the disorder and notes that the stuttering is often accompanied by vocal strain and respiratory gasps. Only for this child, then, would Bloodstein expect the child's stuttering to be influenced by factors such as word length, initial sound of the word, grammatical function, and high "information load."

In 1981 Bloodstein and Grossman found word repetitions occurred the most frequently in the early stuttering of 5 pre-school children. Both word and phrase repetitions occurred consistently at the beginning of syntactic units. Sound and syllable repetitions, prolongations, and hard attacks appeared frequently "in conjunction with word or phrase repetitions as features of the same moment of stuttering." (1981, p. 301). At least some of the sound and syllable repetitions and prolongations indicated difficulty in initiating syntactic units, thus supporting their earlier findings. An earlier study by Bloodstein and Gantwerk (1967) of 13 children ages 2-6 years did not find the typical grammatical effect reported in older children and adults. Any trend that did appear indicated stuttering was more frequent on function words, especially pronouns and conjunctions which also tended to be the first words of these children's clauses or sentences.

Studies by Brown (1945), Williams, Silverman and Kools (1969) and others indicate that the reverse condition occurs in stuttering in older children and adults. The loci of fully developed stuttering depends on attributes of words: more often on words beginning with consonants than with vowels, on content words than function words (although this one finding has been questioned by Soderberg, 1967, and several others), and on polysyllabic than monosyllabic words. Studies by Boomer (1965), Goldman-Eisler (1958), Quarrington (1965), Schlesinger et al (1965), and others on older children and adults show that both stuttering and normal hesitation phenomena are associated with high points of information or with statistical uncertainty in the speech sequence. Boomer (1965) and others had suggested that the encoding unit in speech is a sequence of words and that grammatical and lexical decisions are being made by the speaker. Soderberg (1967) studied the distributions of stuttering and stuttering types of 10 stutterers (ages 9-44). His findings do not support the view that in fully developed stuttering breakdown occurs more on content words. Soderberg hypothesized that stuttering is related primarily to grammatical uncertainty in young children and to both grammatical and lexical uncertainty in advanced stuttering. Soderberg found prolongation tends to occur on lexical words and high information words; repetition tends to occur on function words and low information words. He suggests the possibility that prolongation indicates more difficult decision-making than does repetition. McClay and Osgood (1959) hypothesized that repetitions occur when the speaker needs to delay in order to make a difficult choice.

Bernstein (1981) questioned whether earlier studies provided adequate information about the relationship of sentence-level processing constraints to stuttering on individual words. Her findings for 2 groups of 8 young stuttering children (age preschool through second grade) compared to 8 normally fluent peers generally support the concept of syntactic constraints on the locus of disfluency but for different reasons. Both normal speaking and stuttering children on an elicited language task in Bernstein's study exhibited disfluencies: hesitations, whole word and part-word repetitions, filled pauses, prolonged segments, and revised sentences. The two groups were roughly similar in type and distribution of disfluency. Hesitation was the most frequent type of disfluency for both groups, and hesitation and word-level repetitions occurred significantly oftener than did the other disfluencies for the stutterers. There was a qualitative difference between some of the more tense and extended repetitions of the stuttering children. For both groups, disfluencies occurred oftener on or just prior to the first word of a grammatical unit—chiefly on the initial noun phrases and on the linking conjunction 'and'. Bernstein pointed out that fluency breakdown is expected to occur on the first noun phrase—that is, when initiating the utterance as a whole. Major processing demands are assumed to occur just prior to initiating a sentence. While early associationist models of language conceptualized word by word processing of spoken language, studies of children and adults strongly suggest that processing occurs by the clause. Bernstein found one major difference. The stuttering children were disfluent on the initial word of verb phrases whereas the normal speaking children usually were not.

It seems appropriate to include here information relative to the planning process in reference to producing utterances. Lindsley (1975, 1976) states that adults may begin to utter a sentence before they have processed all the information about the verb such as number agreement with the preceding subject and verb tense. In a later study, also with adults, Lindsley (1976) pointed out that the speaker in uttering a subject phrase has at least a two-syllable delay before he utters the verb which may be sufficient time for him to process information and remain fluent. Bernstein (1981), in applying this information to young stutterers, hypothesizes that children require more time to integrate parts of grammatical units. She suggests it is "levels of strain inherent in planning of syntactic strings" (p. 349) or higher-level sentence planning processes rather than specific word, sound or motor-gesture attributes of the syntactic structures which precipitate fluency breaks. Since normal speaking children also exhibit disfluency and disfluency patterns which she sees as largely congruent with those of stuttering children, she interprets the findings as supportive of the viewpoint that disfluency is a common childhood process, and that it is the manifest form of the disfluency rather than what precipitates it that differentiates the two groups.

Wall (1980) compared the syntactic structure of spontaneous speech utterances of four young male stutterers ranging in age from 5½ years to 6½ matched for age, sex, parental occupation, and birth order with four nonstutterers. Wall found that the stutterers used less complex sentences, fewer complete clauses, more "and" coordinate clauses, and fewer "that" complement clauses. The results suggest that young stutterers may differ from nonstuttering peers in respect to language usage: primarily less efficient and less mature syntax. Whether these young stutterers used simpler, less mature syntax because they stuttered or actually do have some difficulty in constructing sentences on a level with their peers is not known. Wall's study supports Muma's (1971) finding on 13 highly disfluent and 13 highly fluent nonstuttering 4 year olds that disfluent preschool children spoke fewer 'double-based' (complex) sentences than did the fluent children.

Additional information has been obtained through observation reports from clinicians who work with language-delayed children. Hall (1977), Bloodstein (1975), VanRiper (1971) and many clinicians have observed that some school-age children develop episodes of excessive disfluency while receiving articulation and language therapy. Hall (1977) presented case studies of two language-disordered school age children who suddenly became excessively disfluent. As the two children increased their proficiency in language skills, particularly expressive use of syntax, the disfluencies decreased. It was Hall's contention that the development of disfluencies in language-disordered children may be an aspect of normal language acquisition. She stated the clinical observation that children with normally developing language skills become obviously disfluent when they are making great strides linguistically. Hall believes language-disordered children probably experience similar difficulties when they undergo language acquisition remediation.

Actual experimental investigation of the relationship between language delay, language therapy, and disfluency was undertaken by Merits-Patterson and Reed (1981) using matched groups ages 4 to 6. Children in experimental group I were receiving language therapy focusing on increasing mean length of utterance and improving syntactic abilities, while children in experimental group II were not receiving therapy. The control group of 9 children had normal language development. No child was totally fluent. The language-delayed children receiving therapy had more total moments of disfluency and greater variation in total moments than did either the language-delayed nontherapy group or the normal control group. The language-delayed children receiving therapy exhibited more part-word repetitions and whole word repetitions than the other two groups. There were no significant differences in total disfluencies or type of disfluency between the language-delayed nontherapy group and the normal language control group. Merits-Patterson and Reed concluded that for the nontherapy experimental group language delay in itself did not affect fluency. These researchers acknowledge the absence of pre-therapy disfluency data on the language-delayed therapy group. However, they believe the results of the present study suggest language therapy may be related to increased disfluencies.

For the purposes of this chapter it is important to recognize that stutterers with additional disorders do exist. Information on concomitant problems of children who stutter, 14 years and younger, was obtained through a questionnaire survey designed by Blood and Seider (1981). Clinicians from 31 states returned survey data on 1060 stutterers. Of those identified as stutterers, 68% were judged to have other problems. Language disorders and stuttering were present in 10% of the children reported in the survey.

The reader is referred to the research of Riley and Riley

(1979, 1980) for development of a differential diagnostic system through factor analysis of motor and linguistic variables in children who stutter and for conceptualization of a model relating 9 components to the development of stuttering in children. Of relevance to the current topic is Riley and Riley's inclusion of 'sentence formulation difficulties' as one of the four neurologic components. A discussion of the distribution of the components among 54 children and the results of a component based treatment program on 32 of the children is presented in considerable detail in their articles.

There clearly is need for innovative experimental designs, more systematic procedures, and more refined tools in studying the development of disfluency and its relationship to language formulation. We need to be cognizant of the fact that subtle differences in aspects of processing, memory, word retrieval, cognition and formulation may not be readily detected at preschool ages. Our knowledge reflects the status of our current research in the field and is not assumed to be 'the definitive work.' May we continue to investigate creatively and productively!

Assessment Procedures

Our efforts to understand the nature and development of disfluency and stuttering in preschool children are hampered by the fact that the sources of our information—the children—often are not identified when the disfluency first occurs. Typically there is a considerable time lapse between parents' judgment that their child's disfluency is of concern to them or to the child and their decision to contact the staff of a speech and hearing center.

When a very young child is referred for assessment and management of disfluency, we believe every effort should be made to schedule the initial contact within a week following the request. For some children, a single assessment and problem-solving/demonstration management session has been sufficient. Other children have continued in parent-child-clinician management programs. It has been possible to collect data in single-subject studies over several months on specific preschool children. It is that information relative to the children's development of disfluency and development of language production which I wish to share with you.*

---

*Although the pronoun "he" will be used in the discussion, it refers to both males and females.

The children included 15 males and 6 females ages 2 to 4½. Approximately one-third of these children have one parent who is a specialist in speech-language disorders or a related field as learning disabilities or elementary teaching. Eighty percent of the children are enrolled in preschool or kindergarten programs. One-third are involved in lessons for instrumental music, swimming, tumbling, dance or crafts.

During the initial assessment period many parents express concerns about their parenting skills in addition to concerns about the child's disfluency. They frequently volunteer that they have read magazine articles advising them to talk to their children and to ask them questions if they want to increase their child's knowledge and intelligence and help them be 'ready' for school entrance. Educational television programs emphasize knowing colors, shapes, sizes, letters, numbers; counting; reciting the alphabet; and printing your name. Parents often report they are pleased that the child talked early and well. Some report the child said many words at 10 months and talked in sentences at 18 months. Some children tended to follow a more usual timetable for speech and language development. Two had fluctuating hearing losses and at 27 months were considered delayed by their parents.

Parents of some of the 21 children in this study reported that the child had done lots of 'repeating' which was not viewed as a concern. For some, the repeating disappeared for 1 to 2 months and when it returned it was harder, occurred on more words in a sentence and was generally 'worse.' For others, the parents reported excessive repetition with hard stuttering beginning suddenly. They report that the child experienced absolute blockages of air, used a bellowing voice to get words out, exhibited muscle tightness in the mouth area, and switched words. Many of these children were reported initially to continue saying the word until they completed it. As they continued to stutter hard, the children were then observed to prolong initial sounds of words, breaking up phonation and interrupting the air stream. Sometimes pitch rises or gasps for air occurred. Some are reported to have whispered or sung to try to cope with the stuttering.

We ask parents to collect data on the situations in which their child is the most fluent and least fluent. The logs aid in organizing their thinking about the child's speech and in problemsolving throughout the course of therapy. We tell parents that fluency may vary with several aspects of communication including:

1. *the communicative intent:* to direct others, get their attention, ask permission, obtain information, comment,

explain, initiate social interaction;

2. *the competition for a chance to talk and to be listened to;*
3. *the complexity and familiarity of the language formulation:* vocabulary choice, sentence length, plurals, statements vs. questions, pronouns, verb tense, and so forth;
4. *the abstractness of the topic;*
5. *the immediacy of the event:* is it happening here and now;
6. *the excitement level of the situation* or of the child in the situation.

Minor disfluencies in the clinic setting on the day of the evaluation may not be representative of the child's typical fluency levels or pattern. For that reason parents jointly look at a list of disfluent behavior and indicate which ones the child once did or now does. Details about each behavior the parents select are checked against behavior observed during the evaluation. We have grouped the behaviors into the following categories:

DISFLUENCY:

    1. part word and whole word repetition
    2. lengthening of first sound of the word
    3. hesitation before saying a word
    4. can't get the word started

RATE:

    5. fast rate of talking
    6. fast repetitions

BREATHSTREAM:

    7. gasps or quick audible breaths before starting word or between repetitions
    8. cutting off air between repetitions
    9. silent pauses after several repetitions
    10. air wastage—expelling air before utterance begins
    11. speaking at end of breath supply

PHONATION:

    12. hard vocal attacks on the first sound of the word
    13. lengthening of vowels in a word
    14. pitch rise on lengthened vowels
    15. intermittent phonation
    16. vocal fry
    17. tense quality to prolonged vowels

SEQUENCING:

    18. choppy speech or no linking of words within phrases
    19. difficulty in sequencing from one phoneme to another
    20. makes transition from consonant to vowel too slowly
    21. changes in vowel, getting closer approximation (e.g. rah-ruh-rih-ring)

TENSING:
22. forcing through words
23. tension in area around lips with or without lip protrusion
24. tension in jaw
25. tremor
26. body mannerisms as eye blinks or head nodding

ALTERING INTENDED COMMUNICATION:
27. frequent use of "um" or "uh" when the child knows the word he wants to say
28. using vocalized "M" or "N" when the word starts with another sound
29. changing words or abandoning the word and going on to the next sentence
30. rearranging sentences or unexpectedly changing phrase order
31. suddenly switching into singing part of the sentence
32. whispering
33. talking at a higher pitch level
34. increased loudness to get words out

REACTIONS:
35. talking less
36. frustration
37. comments about talking
38. breaking eye contact before or after stuttering
39. crying
40. change in personality—aggressive, withdrawn, etc.

FLUENT PRODUCTIONS:
Certain behaviors in the child's fluent productions signal misuse of the respiratory-phonatory-articulatory system and are of concern:
41. hard vocal attacks
42. hard contacts on the first sound of the word
43. increase in vocal intensity

We gather data on ONSET and DEVELOPMENT of the disfluency, RELATIVES who ever stuttered, PARENTS' REACTIONS and COPING STRATEGIES. Observation and audio tape recording is done during parent-child interactions and clinician-child interactions. Often one parent observes through the two-way mirror and the clinician can ask questions to clarify parents' reporting.

Initially the parent is encouraged to interact in a typical manner. During the parent-child interaction parents have been observed to ask numerous questions of the child, speak at a rapid rate, talk in long sentences, give complex instructions, and use vocabulary difficult for a child to produce. Much of parents' communicative intent appears to be to direct behavior, to display the child's knowledge, to checkout what a child knows and understands, and to teach. Careful observation is made of changes in form and frequency of the child's stuttering as communicative pressure and interaction style are systematically varied. Typical conditions observed include: highly exciting activity, adult talking quickly, adult asking many questions, adult speaking in long complex sentences, adult directing the activity or asking about an earlier event.

After making these observations, the clinician models desired interaction changes and notes changes in the child's speech. If a reduction in severity or frequency occurs, the behavioral change is pointed out to the parent, the strategies are explained and demonstrated, and the parent invited to interact with the child as the clinician 'coaches' them through the procedures.

If fluency building strategies of modeling simpler language patterns said at a slow rate together with reduction of fluency disruptors is effective during the evaluation session, then these strategies are likely to be effective when done by the parents at home. Modeling simpler language patterns at a slower rate has been most effective with children at *early* stages of language development. Although age is not the criterion, most of the children in this category are 3-0 or younger. Parents of these children often are able to modify verbal interaction style quickly, particularly when they discover that their manner of talking has a direct effect on the child's fluency. The parents want to know what they can do themselves and find their success reinforcing. About half of these parents feel comfortable implementing the strategies on their own. The clinician keeps contact by telephone and arranges to see the child immediately if stuttering increases or the pattern changes. Other parents prefer that the clinician work jointly with them and the child for 3 to 10 sessions. The parents' need for continued guidance and support may cease in 3 sessions or continue for 6 to 9 months.

If the child's stuttering when it occurs is judged to be moderately severe, even though the child speaks fluently 50% or more of the time during the evaluation session, it is doubtful that fluency building strategies alone will be sufficient. Although age is not the criterion here either, many of the children in this category are ages 3-0 to 4-0. We expect to do a little direct altering of the child's talking behavior particularly in regard to teaching gentle phonation and reducing effort and muscle tension in the laryngeal area and abdominal area.

Early Intervention and Prevention of Stuttering
Guidelines for Verbal Interaction

It has been found effective during adult-child verbal interactions to reduce the excitement level of activities, for parents and others to talk at a slower rate, to reduce the number of questions, and to program some silent periods during play. Examinations of tape recordings show that this type of parent-child interaction does alter the frequency and type of disfluencies, length of child's utterances, rate of child's speech, and audible characteristics of effort associated with disfluencies. The following are guidelines for strategies that parents can implement aimed toward encouraging children to verbalize at a less stressful level linguistically. As we work with parents, we discuss with them our joint efforts to implement the strategies and we engage in problem solving discussions.

1. RATE. One factor that may affect fluency is the rate at which the child and those around him talk. Often children try to talk fast to keep pace with the adult's rate of speech. When children hurry, especially if they are only 2 or 3 or 4 years old, they may repeat and hesitate because their tongues, lips, and jaws simply cannot move that quickly. There is a greater likelihood of incoordination of breathing, voicing and sound formation at a fast rate. Once a child has learned to talk rapidly it is often harder to talk more slowly later on. Some youngsters become programmed for hurrying. If we reduce our own rate of talking a little, then the youngster may learn to talk slower also. It may be helpful to verbalize that "he doesn't have to hurry because Mother and Dad have time to listen." However, people should not tell a child to "slow down—take your time." Such advice may give him the idea that he is doing something wrong when he talks and that he should try not to talk as he does now. In his attempt to stop doing that "something wrong" his muscles may stiffen and the disfluencies may increase.

As some children become more involved in activities they talk faster and their speech, though fluent, is less clear. When they become even more excited, some of their speech is not intelligible. The rate is so fast that words are jumbled together, sounds slurred, and syllables seem omitted. Children who speak super fast may repeat the initial word or part of it and repeat linking words such as "and" to give themselves time to formulate ideas.

2. QUESTIONS. Young children's disfluencies have been observed to increase if we ask them many questions. Much of adults' verbal communication with children is question-asking in nature. Questions put children on the spot for a response. We believe that sometimes it will be helpful to change the verbal interaction style with a child to reduce the number of questions, for example, try to reduce by 50 percent the number of questions asked. Parents have found it helpful to do more "commenting." The commenting strategy involves verbalizing in short sentences what the parent thinks the child is doing, feeling and thinking as he is playing or being with them; it's a little like saying thoughts aloud.

3. DISPLAY SPEECH. It is important not to put children on the spot in another way. Avoid doing the "Show and Tell" routine. It is disruptive of thought processes, requires a great deal of memory, and puts too much attention on the child's language formulation skills, for example, to direct him: "Tell Daddy where he went;" "Tell Mommy who we saw;" "Tell Grandpa what you got for your birthday," etc. An adult can comment and give information about the event to Dad, Mother, or Grandfather. If the child wants to chime in and add his own comments, fine.

4. HERE AND NOW. Young children's fluency often increases if we make use of the idea of the "here and now." Children have been observed to be more fluent and to acquire a vocabulary of labels faster when the object or event being talked about is right in front of them. If a child has to recall what was done or seen yesterday or an hour ago, he appears to search more for the word names and for the words to express thoughts. The object's actual physical presence seems to facilitate verbalization. A substitute for the object is a picture book. When looking at a picture book together or reading a story, refrain from quizzing about the pictures. Instead of asking "What's this?" or "Do dogs have tails?" name some of the pictures or features of the picture or comment on the action. If the child wants to name pictures spontaneously or comment on them, then this is less stressful and more conducive to better fluency.

5. ECHOING. For very young children, less than 3 years old, disfluencies may decrease if we sometime echo part of what they have just said rather than engage in a conversation. One caution, if the child stutters, simply echo fluently what he said without calling attention to the stuttering. It is not an exciting way to talk with a child but it can provide an awareness that we have understood. A child relaxes and enjoys talking when he feels the

message is getting through to the listener. Further, the child does not feel the adult will take over the conversation and change the topic. It is suggested that only the parents do some echoing and that they plan to stop the echoing gradually in one to two months. However, if the child responds negatively to the echoing or considers such to be teasing, stop doing it immediately.

6. LISTENING AND ATTENDING. Children's disfluencies may increase when they want us to listen to them. They are not good at waiting their turn. Often, to gain attention, they interrupt our talking to someone or interrupt our activity. Many young children want us to look at them and want to be able to see our eyes when they talk. They do not want us to continue preparing a meal or reading as we listen. They seem to want 100 percent of our attention. If it isn't possible to give undivided attention at that moment, ask them to wait a minute. We may expect a child to speak with more disfluencies when the parents are involved in another task, e.g., focusing on driving a car. Parents cannot turn to look at the child very much at that time. In addition, the youngster may experience more disfluency because he wants to call your attention to something which is rapidly disappearing from view as you drive by.

Children may begin a verbal interaction with a person's name, as "Mom," repeated 3 to 10 times. The remainder of the sentence may be fluent. What you do depends on whether the repetition of "Mom" is a signal: "Hey, listen" or whether it is said to give him time to organize his thoughts before verbalizing them aloud.

7. LANGUAGE DEVELOPMENT. For some children ages 2 to 4 years, the disfluencies appear to be due, at least in part, to their stage of language development. They are learning new words and linking them together in sentences. They are learning to ask questions that require a different word order than do sentences. Their expressive language and comprehension are expanding. Thus, children are often more disfluent at this stage of vocabulary acquisition and language formulation. Our goal is to reduce language development pressure. We believe it is helpful for adults to decrease markedly their efforts to teach vocabulary labels, concepts, colors, printing, etc. for 2 to 3 months. The child will not stop learning but he may learn at a more relaxed pace. Once more normal fluency has been reestablished, parents can return to the teaching activities. Parents can enjoy being with a child without trying to "teach" or "direct," such as when engaged in table top crafts or sand box activities. The activity should be one that lends itself to 'doing' without feeling a need

to talk constantly. Leave more PAUSE TIME when you talk, spaces where the child can insert his ideas if he wishes or spaces where both of you are comfortable with silence. Some parents have actually programmed 'quiet' time or 'thinking' time. If, however, the child feels he is losing his turn during the waiting period, this strategy will fail. Teach "turn taking" if the disfluencies increase when the child wants to take command of the situation and wants to refocus the attention on himself.

Talk in simple, short sentences. Break longer sentences into phrase groups, pausing briefly between them. It's like chunking a telephone number. If we observe that a child is fluent when he talks in short phrases (3-4 words), this is a clue that sentence length is important in the maintaining of fluency.

We believe some children may be disfluent because motorically they are attempting to coordinate respiratory, phonatory and articulatory systems at a level above their physical capability. We also believe that the greater the uncertainty about information, the longer and more complex the sentence formulation, and the greater the number of linguistic decisions to be made, the more likely it is that coordination will be disrupted and disfluency occur.

More Specific Fluency Building Strategies

There are many children regardless of age whose stuttering severity can be altered little by the clinician during the evaluation. It may also be apparent that environmental manipulation and altering of interaction styles will be less effective and that direct altering of the child's talking behavior is needed. It is likely, too, that the parents and clinician will need to problem-solve in nearly every therapy session for strategies that will reduce the severity of the stuttering. Three behaviors signal a need for direct intervention: (1) breath stream mismanagement and/or hard vocal attacks; (2) active attempts to stop stuttering; (3) active attempts to conceal stuttering.

The clinician devises tasks that are appropriate for a child 2—4½ years of age in terms of motor coordination, comprehension, and conceptualization. We do not focus on stuttering. As much as possible, the clinician models the easier production on single words giving appropriate instructions to start words easily with lips just barely touching.

Very little understanding of what to do can be grasped from verbal directions by children 2½ to 4½ years old. Many children do not want to follow your 'lead' even when playing a "Copy Me" game. They can be highly independent. At times, clinicians can get a preschool child to say words in unison through a demonstration of "Watch my mouth" and instructions to "Say it with me." It is not effective to ask an independent, sensitive child to "Say it *over*, easy." Usually they refuse and refuse to continue working with you. A wiser strategy is to say, "Do the next one super easy" and *model* for the child the behavior you want. We comment on how the child can be the "boss of his mouth" and "talk easy." We do not ask preschool children to try "easy" and "hard" versions of a word. Usually children try too hard and become blocked and frightened when they cannot utter the word. One difficulty with a young child is that of finding strategies which can be done through game approaches but enable the clinician to have some control over the kind of talking being done by the child. When a child senses he has a hard time talking he is more willing to say words or talk in a manner directed by the clinician. When there is even the slightest improvement, the child decides "his talking is fixed now" and he would rather play freely with the toys. However, the clinician should continue some work on the strategies suggested below to ensure that the more fluent speech continues and that the child comes to perceive himself as enjoying talking and being successful. For any of the suggested strategies, if the child will do them for 3 to 5 minutes each, the clinician is pleased.

When the program detailed below is recommended, we explain to parents that their child has stuttered too many months and that his pattern of laryngeal closure and breathstream mismanagement seems too well learned to be reduced or eliminated simply by removing pressures. It is explained that talking is a complex behavior and that their child is not doing certain aspects of the process in a way to facilitate fluent talking. We discuss the talking process with parents and work on specific aspects that the child is mismanaging. A summary of the program and some rationale follows:

1. RATE. We need to devise games to say words or phrases slowly. Obtain 15 - 25 words said slowly if possible. We doubt that the child will detect that the clinician is talking slowly, so he will need to be asked to talk slower and to have it demonstrated for him. We do not want to create "choppy" speech if he talks in phrases or sentences, so it is necessary to *link* words together. Slower rate reduces the number of repetitions per word and increases the chances of obtaining easier vocal onset.

2. INTENSITY. We need to devise a game in which all the players talk *softly*. Perhaps the child can talk in his typically

formulated phrases and sentences but softly—as if what we say is in our "little voice" vs. our "big voice," or "inside voice" vs. "outside voice," or "quiet voice" vs. "loud voice." Many times when young children try to talk quietly the only thing they can do is to whisper. At this stage and time such is acceptable. We do not want a "loud whisper" effect since such may increase muscle effort and physical tension in the larynx and diaphragm. If there is laryngeal tension beyond the amount desired, then talking softly and gently and slowly is likely to result in short repeated blockings or hard repetitions rather than hard blockages with the air shut off, and we judge that to be an improvement. If the blockings are short or if he only repeats, we have observed clinically that the child is less likely to switch words or rearrange his sentences. He is more likely to continue saying the intended word and to be affected less by the stuttering when it occurs. Again this is judged as progress. We can increase the possibilities of more adequate laryngeal functioning by the words selected for the child to say.

3. PHONATORY REQUIREMENTS. We need to be concerned with the effect of voiceless and voiced sounds, and with laryngeal functioning for "onset" and "termination" of voicing within words. Many children demonstrate more severe stuttering whenever they say a word that begins with a vowel or a diphthong. Sometimes they cannot initiate words beginning with stops: for example, "key" or "puppy." We have to experiment more with words to be certain of clinical hunches, but based on experience we expect a child to be more fluent on words beginning with voiced continuants. Examples include words such as "mama," "wagon," perhaps even "rabbit" or "zipper." A child is expected to have more difficulty on words beginning with voiceless continuants such as "five" or "some" since there is a switch from voiceless "f" to voiced "i" and from voiceless "s" to voiced "o." We do not think it wise to tell a child that he has a hard time saying words beginning with the letter "i" or "k," etc. It is acceptable to tell him—if he seems concerned—that some words may be easier to say and that we will help him change his talking on the harder words.

4. BREATHING AND BREATH STREAM MANAGEMENT. Taking a deep breath and holding it, shutting off air in the throat or mouth, gasping, speaking without sufficient breath, or talking long 'run-on' sentences are some of the behaviors we have observed. It may be difficult for children to control the breath stream. We devise games in which he can experience relaxed breathing and a return to normal breathing pattern. To begin

with, we try activities that do not require talking. For example, the parent, the child, and the clinician can lie on their backs on the floor—just relaxing, certainly not "resting for sleep." We can look at the ceiling and just breathe in and out easily—no forcing, no altering of the normal pattern. When we are relaxed, we can exhale the air gently—just the tiniest amount, by turn. The clinician models for the child and the parent. The clinician can take a turn, then the parent, then the child. Then we can take turns at being a "little wind" and make an "oooooooo" sound. If the child is willing, the clinician can say a number or a word, then the child, etc., with one word per exhaled breath at the start. We can aim for phrases and short sentences later. A similarly effective strategy for keeping air stream and phonation continuous involves a game in which the child and the parent move turtles slowly over a road. The road can be drawn on brown paper and needs to have a hill so that we can demonstrate sliding easily down the hill and moving slowly on the road. We can slide a sound or a word said in slow motion. The idea is to make all the sounds in the word slightly more slowly. It is incorrect to stretch the first sound or the vowel of the word only.

5. EFFORT AND MUSCLE TENSION. Sometimes a child seems to be forcing words out. His abdomen and chest are very rigid or tensed. He will not know what to do if he is directed to "relax." It can be effective with some children for the clinician to rub their "tummy" very very lightly and say "Keep your tummy soft" as you rub.

6. RHYTHM. If he likes singing, we can sing with real words or silly syllables. Try clapping hands to get a timing effect without singing, or beating on a plastic bowl with wooden spoons as we say words or phrases. It is important to use a *variety* of rhythmic timers rather than just one. We can play drums with syllables as "wah—wah-wah-wah" and perhaps the first "wah" can be stressed slightly more.

7. ATTITUDE. It is important for the child to hear us say, when it is appropriate to the situation, that we *learn* to talk and when we learn we sometimes make mistakes. It's no big deal. We can fix mistakes. And, a mistake is not "bad." This implies that the parents and clinician need to remove as much as possible the *value* words from their verbal interaction with a child. We need to omit words such as "right," "wrong," "good," "bad," "nice" and instead, praise for "ideas he has to share" and "for interesting pictures he drew." He also needs to feel that we believe he won't always talk hard and that we can help him change his talking. Perhaps none of the above ideas will work as effectively as

we wish. Then we will continue to problem-solve together for other strategies.

In today's culture, many families try to be open in respect to feelings and in other areas of living. Yet they have been advised to ignore stuttering and avoid dealing verbally with the fact that it occurs. Parents notice bruises, dirty hands, torn clothing. A child may expect a parent to notice when he has difficulty talking. And he may expect the parent to *help* him talk. After all, parents bandage cuts, attend to stomach aches, repair bicycles. Why don't they get his talking fixed? Children cry, act out, and verbally acknowledge their concern. Direct quotes from children include: "You be the Indian Chief who doesn't like the way I talk." "I have trouble with my h-h-h." "The doctor forgot to check my words." There is no need to ignore disfluencies that are of concern to a child. A parent can calmly comment, "Yes, some times it may be harder to talk. But it won't always be. There are people who know how to help you talk." Clinicians and parents can intervene to reduce fluency disruptors, to build fluency skills, and to alter stuttering behavior in preschool children.

References

Bernstein, N., "Are There Constraints on Childhood Disfluency?", *Journal of Fluency Disorders*, 6, 341-350, 1981.

Blood, G., and Seider, R., "The Concomitant Problems of Young Stutterers," *Journal of Speech and Hearing Disorders*, 46, 31-33, 1981.

Bloodstein, O., *A Handbook on Stuttering*. Chicago, Illinois, National Easter Seal Society for Crippled Children and Adults, 1975.

Bloodstein, O., "The Rules of Early Stuttering," *Journal of Speech and Hearing Disorders*, 39, 379-394, 1974.

Bloodstein, O., and Gantwerk, B., "Grammatical Function in Relation to Stuttering in Young Children," *Journal of Speech and Hearing Research*, 10, 787-789, 1967.

Bloodstein, O., and Grossman, M., "Early Stutterings: Some Aspects of Their Form and Distribution," *Journal of Speech and Hearing Research*, 24, 298-302, 1981.

Boomer, D., "Hesitation and Grammatical Encoding," *Language and Speech*, 8, 148-158, 1965.

Brown, S., "The Loci of Stuttering in the Speech Sequence," *Journal of Speech Disorders*, 10, 181-192, 1945.

Goldman-Eisler, F., "The Predictability of Words in Context and the Length of Pauses in Speech," *Language and Speech*, 1, 226-231, 1958.

Hall, P., "The Occurrence of Disfluencies in Language-disordered School-age Children," *Journal of Speech and Hearing Disorders*, 42, 364-369, 1977.

Lindsley, J., "Producing Simple Utterances: How Far Ahead Do We Plan?", *Cognitive Psychology*, 7, 1-19, 1975.

Lindsley, J., "Producing Simple Utterances: Details of the Planning Process," *Journal of Psycholinguistic Research*, 5, 331-353, 1976.

McClay, H., and Osgood, C., "Hesitation Phenomena in Spontaneous English Speech," *Word*, 15, 19-44, 1959.

Merits-Patterson, R., and Reed, C., "Disfluencies in the Speech of Language-disordered Children," *Journal of Speech and Hearing Research*, 46, 55-58, 1981.

Muma, J., "Syntax of Preschool Fluent and Dysfluent Speech: A Transformational Analysis," *Journal of Speech and Hearing Research*, 14, 428-441, 1971.

Pearl, S., and Bernthal, J., "The Effect of Grammatical Complexity Upon Disfluency Behavior of Nonstuttering Preschool Children," *Journal of Fluency Disorders*, 5, 55-68, 1980.

Quarrington, B., "Stuttering as a Function of the Information Value and Sentence Position of Words," *Journal of Abnormal Psychology*, 70, 221-224, 1965.

Riley, G., and Riley, J., "A Component Model for Diagnosing and Treating Children Who Stutter," *Journal of Fluency Disorders*, 4, 279-293, 1979.

Riley, G., and Riley, J., "Motoric and Linguistic Variables Among Children Who Stutter," *Journal of Speech and Hearing Disorders*, 45, 504-514, 1980.

Schlesinger, I., Forte, M., Fried, B. and Melkman, R., "Stuttering, Information Load, and Response Strength," *Journal of Speech and Hearing Disorders*, 30, 32-36, 1965.

Slobin, D., "Grammatical Transformation and Sentence Comprehension in Childhood and Adulthood," *Journal of Verbal Learning and Verbal Behavior*, 5, 219-227, 1966.

Soderberg, G., "Linguistic Factors in Stuttering," *Journal of Speech and Hearing Research*, 10, 801-810, 1967.

VanRiper, C., *The Nature of Stuttering*. Englewood Cliffs, New Jersey, Prentice-Hall, 1971.

Wall, M., "A Comparison of Syntax in Young Stutterers and Non-stutterers," *Journal of Fluency Disorders*, 5, 345-352, 1980.

Williams, D., Silverman, F., and Kools, J., "Disfluency Behavior of Elementary-school Stutterers and Nonstutterers: Loci of Instances of Disfluencies," *Journal of Speech and Hearing Research*, 12, 308-318, 1969.

chapter three

Speech Motor Processes and Stuttering in Children; A Theoretical and Clinical Perspective

John M. Hanley, Ph.D.
Western Michigan University

Many variables (genetic, physiological, psychological, linguistic, emotional, and learning) have been associated with the problem of stuttering. Some of these variables may be more relevant than others, not necessarily as "causal" elements, but as significant components of the communicative experience. However, until we are better able to relate these variables to the physiological processes or mechanisms underlying speech production, we can only view them as "associated conditions" that *may* contribute to the breakdown of speech motor processes and that should be considered in therapy.

Recently, Zimmermann, Smith and Hanley (1980) proposed a theoretical perspective or framework for stuttering that may unify the segmented efforts and vocabularies of those working in the research areas of speech science, physiology, linguistics, and psychology. We proposed that several types of events occur at various levels of the speech production system or the communicative environment. We suggested that learning, physiological, psychological, linguistic, and genetic variables all play a potentially important role in the breakdown of speech coordination and the perceived disfluencies that result. However, the relevance of any of these variables cannot be understood until they can be described in terms of their effect on the alteration of motor neuron pools that effect coordinated or discoordinated speech movements. The incorporation of such a framework requires that research efforts and clinical strategies relate these linguistic, learning, or psychological variables thought to be important to the processes and principles of operation of the neurophysiological system.

It is possible that many of these pertinent psychological, linguistic, or emotional events have similar effects on the neuromotor system, e.g., they will contribute directly or indirectly to the alteration of neuromotor activity resulting in discoordinated speech movements. Also, the effect of various therapeutic procedures (desensitization, prolonged speech, easy voicing, relaxation, etc.) may be very similar when considered in terms of the neurophysiological adjustments which emerge from such procedures. Therapies may differ in their efficacy, but the neurophysiological adjustments that result from each may be very similar.

This framework does not imply causality. Rather, it encourages us to consider stuttering as a product of dynamic interactions of variables at various levels of the speech production system. Some of these variables may be more relevant than others, not necessarily as "causal" elements, but as significant components of the communicative experience. Such a perspective is supported by the work of theorists and researchers working in the area of movement physiology, who advocate an "ecological" view of movement control (Johnston and Turvey, 1982; Shettlesworth, 1982; Zimmermann and Kelso, 1983). They suggest that an understanding of motor processes and the malfunction of those processes will emerge from study of the dynamic interplay of organismic and environmental variables. Consideration of the child, his actions, or his environment in any discreet or isolated way may be experimentally or clinically wasteful. The discussion that follows incorporates this perspective into the development of a clinical intervention approach for children who are experiencing problems with fluency.

Intervention: An Individualized Search
for Significant Conditions
and Modification Strategies

Each child who experiences a fluency problem must be considered as a unique individual. On a large variety of continua, they will perform, think, react, or interact in very original ways. Each experience will be novel to some degree, and the "originality" of every communicative activity should be considered as a dynamic experience, part of an organismic-environmental process which generates communicative phenomena, external and internal. When the child's characteristics are considered discreetly, they may be perceived as shy, withdrawn, aggressive, reactive, sensitive, confident, or insecure. Their language development may be precocious or delayed. Their fine and gross motor abilities may be advanced or deficient. Likewise, their parents, siblings, and fellow communicators will be represented by a variety of traits. They may be supportive, shy, expectant, hurried, punative, comfortable, coordinated, anxious, or assertive. The list of individual differences and characteristics could continue for many pages, but the examples listed should be sufficient to suggest that every child, normally fluent or not, possesses unique characteristics and interacts with fellow communicators and environmental situations in a very original and dynamic fashion.

The speech disruptions which characterize the child's communicative behavior will also vary with different situations, with changes of the child's emotional state, with changes of linguistic variables, vocabulary, etc. We do not yet understand the exact reasons for this variability, nor do we understand the relationship between part-word repetitions, prolongations, tense blockages and other perceptible disfluencies and the physiological processes that generate them. Several researchers have established various guidelines for differentiating those disfluencies which are typically judged to be normal or abnormal. Examples of such guidelines may be found in most texts related to the topic of stuttering (e. g. VanRiper, 1982), and the clinician may find such guidelines to be useful *estimates* of typical or atypical behavior. We should recognize, however, that such guidelines are controversial because the physiological and psychological processes which underlie the production of disfluency, typical or atypical, are not yet understood. At the present time, we can only hypothesize about such processes, and it seems reasonable to assume that our best hypotheses may be generated when we consider the occurrence of disfluent behavior in the context of other psychological, emotional, and environmental variables which comprise the child's communicative behavior.

The clinician who encounters the young "atypically" disfluent child may be confused by the "uniqueness" of his personality, his disfluencies, and other aspects of his communicative behavior. The clinician may feel the need to describe at the beginning the "best" or "most ideal" therapy program for a particular child. However, more clinicians are coming to understand that the present status of our knowledge of the variables involved in stuttering provides only general guidelines, and that in working with each child and his parents the unique characteristics contributing to the problem need to be observed and evaluated. Likewise, therapy procedures must be assessed and adjusted to meet the evolving objectives of the therapeutic process. The following discussion is based upon such an individualized, descriptive, experimental perspective.

Initiation of the Clinical Experience

The initial interactions with the child and his parents are very important. During this time, we have the opportunity to discuss current perspectives and controvercies surrounding the onset and development of speech disorders. We begin to gather data concerning the child, his speech, his communicative behavior, and aspects of his environment that will form the basis for the development of hypotheses regarding procedural decisions and client/parent/clinician discussions that will emerge. Based upon the unifying theoretical perspective described earlier (Zimmermann, Smith, and Hanley, 1980) and upon current hypotheses of movement control (Zimmermann and Kelso, 1983; Kelso, Tuller, and Harris, 1983) the following considerations or assumptions seem reasonable as a basis for a clinical perspective and as topics for presentation and discussion with parents and children:

1. We do not yet completely understand the operation of the normal speech production system or the motor control mechanisms that function to effect fluent or disfluent speech production.

2. We have developed a number of speculative theories, interpretations, and therapy approaches that are based upon genetic, physiological, psychodynamic, learning, linguistic, and environmental variables as "causal" elements underpinning fluency or disfluency. The validity of those perspectives has not been fully determined.

42

3. We have measured and observed a vast number of genetic, behavioral, psychodynamic, linguistic, and environmental variables that appear to be correlated with fluent or disfluent speech. The mechanisms of these associations has not yet been determined.
4. We have not yet discovered a specific set of activities or variables that will insure the recovery of the child or insure the development of *normal* fluency and communication.
5. Based upon the high degree of variability of fluency behavior, emotionality, and environmental events within and across children who experience fluency problems, we can only assume that the significant events or conditions associated with fluency breakdown must be determined on an individual basis. Parents should also be advised that, to the best of our knowledge, the etiologic "formula" for speech breakdown may not be the same for all stutterers, in all situations, or at different stages of development of the disorder.
6. Current movement control theory suggests that the interaction of a number of different variables (genetic, physiological, social, linguistic, psychological) rather than the action of any particular discreet variable may be critical for the instigation of breakdown of the motor processes underlying stuttering.
7. The most efficient and meaningful management procedures may vary across individuals, situations, or developmental stages of the problem.
8. In individual children, variables typically classified as emotional, linguistic, environmental, psychological, or physiological may require adjustment to reestablish or maintain conditions conducive to fluency.

Taken together, these assumptions imply that the most fruitful, efficient, and meaningful clinical activities for the child may be determined only if we undertake a careful, ongoing, descriptive approach toward the development of a management program (Zimmermann and Hanley, 1982). These assumptions also imply that a meaningful management program should be somewhat experimental in nature, i.e., the treatment program should include a careful description of events, the development of hypotheses about significant events that must be altered, and a selection of techniques designed to test our hypotheses (i.e. behavior modification, counseling, modeling-imitation, etc.).

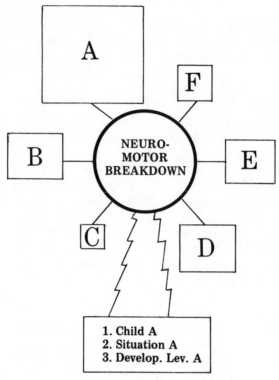

FIGURE 1
Example of Variables Affecting Neuro-motor Breakdown

A Clinical Framework

As a framework for the clinical experience with the child and parent, we may assume that an undetermined "formula," comprised of different types of variables, determines the physiological breakdown we perceive as stuttering. As emphasized above, these "significant" variables may differ in quantity or quality for different individuals and for different communicative settings. In fact, we recognize the possibility that a number of "formulae" may exist for each child, for different types of communicative settings, and for different stages of development of the problem.

As a mechanism for enhancing the parent's (or child's) conceptualization of this perspective, we might portray the motoric breakdown of speech as being comprised of a number of ingredients. The correct combination of ingredients or the amount of each ingredient may form a "recipe" for the child's disfluent experience, and different "recipes" may define motoric breakdown in different settings. A "recipe" model defining the inter-

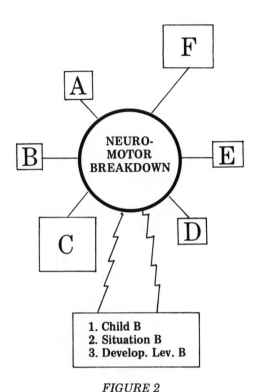

FIGURE 2

*Example of Variables Affecting Neuro-motor Breakdown Illustrating a
Different "Recipe" Compared to the One in Figure 1*

action of different types of variables might be elucidated for the
child or parent by use of metaphorical examples. The 5-6 year
old child may easily recognize that many combinations of ingredients may be used to make a bread recipe "taste good." They
will also recognize that one recipe tastes good on one day and
not on another. They will understand that different recipes
"taste good" for some people and not for others, etc. Motor
activities such as playing a musical instrument or participating
in a sport such as golf may also be used to help a parent understand the dynamic interaction of variables which contribute to
motor proficiency. Anyone familiar with the sport of golf will
understand that coordination, practice, fear of water hazards,
extreme competition, "specific club fears," and the number of
interested observers may all be significant events or ingredients
of breakdown for certain individuals or in certain situations. A
"best" remedial program for a golf swing must take into consideration each of those variables as they interact dynamically.
A visual display, such as the ones presented in Figures 1 and 2

may also be utilized to enhance conceptualization of perspective described.

The size of the boxes in each figure represent the relative contribution of each individually significant variable (A, B, C, etc.) to the breakdown formula. For illustrative purposes, we might conceivably list a set of interactive variables such as the following:

A= A child's perception of listener discomfort

B= A "threshold" of emotional sensitivity or reactivity

C= The linguistic complexity of the child's speech/language behavior

D= A speech characteristic of the listener (i.e., a "hurried" speech delivery which may serve as an inappropriate model for the child to imitate)

E= The complexity of the communicative setting (i.e., communication in a disruptive classroom setting or at a noisy football field)

F= The specific neuromuscular capabilities or limitations of the child at a given time or for a particular situation.

The events or ingredients may differ qualitatively or quantitatively for each of the two "recipes" presented, but both recipes are sufficient to promote speech motor breakdown. Several combinations of factors, then, may interact to promote neuromotor activity which exceeds a critical threshold for breakdown. The figures may represent recipes for two different children, for one child in two different speaking situations, or for one child at two different developmental levels (of stuttering or of physiological development).

Such a conceptual model seems reasonable from a therapeutic as well as from a theoretical standpoint. It is consonant with current perspectives of movement control, coordination, and perception in animals and in humans. It also promotes open-minded, objective consideration of many types of communicative events as being potentially relevant. We can view the diagnostic category of stuttering as a communication problem comprised of several heritable, psychological, physiological, environmental, and linguistic characteristics.

From models such as the one described, we might assume that the success or failure of a communicative experience may involve the dynamic interplay of physiological events (neural, muscle, movement, coordinative) and the acoustic signals which emerge from them, psychological variables (attitudes, fears, emotions, anxieties, personality traits), and psychosocial dynamics (linguistic, nonverbal, listener behavior, and setting). The child's ability to produce coordinated (or fluent) speech movements with different individuals and in different settings may be altered by his unique perceptual experiences, his basic capability to perform speech motor tasks, and the various communicative interactions that develop in different environmental contexts. It may be inappropriate to assume that speech motorics are more important or "causal" than the child's ongoing perceptions, linguistic performance, or other relevant events in his environment. This frame of reference requires that we carefully observe the child's verbal (speech motoric and linguistic) and nonverbal behaviors, his perceptions of his listeners and his environment, and the events (speech and nonspeech) characterizing the behaviors of other communicators in his environment. As we begin to describe these events we should recognize that the events associated with fluency or fluency breakdown may be different (but possibly no less valid) than those being subjected to speculation and investigation in research laboratories and that some of those events may be indirectly modifiable by adjustment of associated events.

Conditions Associated with Fluency Disruptions

The following discussion focuses on the perceptual, physiological, linguistic, and environmental conditions that may be related to disruption of the motoric flow of speech. As previously pointed out in the recipe model, each of these variables may be relevant only in the sense that it is one of several conditions interacting in a communicative experience.

Perceptual Considerations

How often have we read about or experienced a client who reported that his fluent speech experiences were preceded or accompanied by feelings of confidence, of "being relaxed," of feeling comfortable, feelings of "letting it all go," etc.? Those feelings are somehow related to the individual's perceptions of his past experiences, of his current physiological and psychological "state," and, of his physical setting and listeners. Similarly, how often have we had perceptions of the stutterer as "anxious," "hurried," and "hesitant"; or of his listeners as "punitive," "impatient," "uncomfortable," "unattentive," or "bored"? We, the child, and other communicators perceive these and other characteristics frequently. We should recognize that one, or several of the events associated with such perceptions, whether

47

they are part of the child's behavior, the listener's behavior, or the communicative environment, may require clinical attention.

Events that are perceptually relevant for the child may play an extremely important role in the onset and development of fluency problems, yet they may receive little or no attention in the clinical experience. Zimmermann and Hanley (1982) have suggested that the child's perceptions, possibly very different from ours, may determine which events or characteristics of his parents or his environment will be selected for imitation or emotional reaction. Some events will signify success or failure for the child, and others will be associated with fear, comfort, or pain. Those events are likely to be perceived differently by the clinician or parent. Each child may also experience unique perceptions of events as they occur in different communicative settings, or as the style and content of an interaction changes. As part of the communicative network, we should also be aware that those events (i.e., speech characteristics of the child) that are perceptually relevant for the parent may contribute to parent responses (i.e., parent speech or nonverbal behaviors) that are perceptually relevant for the child. The "interaction" hypothesis of Johnson (1959), though developed from a different perspective, suggested that such perceptions and reactions may play a very important role in the onset of stuttering. It seems reasonable, for example, to suspect that a parent who perceives her child as "helpless" during a moment of disfluency may react (often nonverbally) in a fashion that is perceived as "frightened" by the child. If this percept is "relevant" for that child, it may contribute to inappropriate neurological adjustments that promote disfluency. A brief verbal interchange between a 6 year old child and his clinician may illustrate the importance of the child's perceptions and the events related to those perceptions as conditions associated with speech motor breakdown:

Clinician: When you stutter, what do people say that makes you stutter more?
Child:　　"Slow down!"
Clinician: Who says that to you?
Child:　　My dad.
Clinician: Does your mother ever say "Slow down!" after you stutter?
Child:　　Yes.
Clinician: Do you stutter more then?
Child:　　No.
Clinician: Why?
Child:　　. . . cause she's not mad at my talking.

Clinician: You don't stutter more when I tell you to slow down. Why do you think that is?

Child: . . . cause you're trying to help me get better.

The discussion continued, and the clinician hypothesized that when the child perceived someone as trying to be helpful, he became more fluent. A more detailed discussion of his father's behavior indicated that the child perceived his father to be "excited" and disapproving ("He doesn't like me when I do that!") when he stuttered. The clinician advised the child's father of his child's perceptions and their correlation to speech breakdown. He was advised that it may not be "what he said" but "how he said it." The parent responded by attempting to be more "encouraging" and "supportive" in his responses. Within a short time, a noticeable reduction of disfluency was observed during subsequent parent/father interactions. The exact changes of other events or variables is not known. However, the child's subsequent discussions of his father's behavior indicated that the elimination of one perceptually relevant condition ("excited" or "disapproving" father) was fluency enhancing. Another child may ignore "excited" reactions to his speech, and instead perceive his mother's attempts (to be supportive) as a patronizing reaction. In this case, a "patronizing" event may become a condition associated with fluency breakdown. The clinician or parent who is concerned with the prevention of stuttering in the young child should undertake careful description of communicative interactions such as those described above. From such descriptions, they might formulate hypothesis about the interactions of the child's perception of listeners, his perception of their speech behavior, their conversational topics or his perceptions of other characteristics of the conversational environments (settings) which may be correlated with fluency or disfluency. Modification of one or several of those described behaviors, events, perceptions or settings which correlate with motoric breakdown may induce a higher level of fluency in the child's speech. Similarly, early instatement of those events or settings which promote perceptions which are fluency enhancing (i.e., those which are perceived as comfortable, simple, etc.) may promote the interaction of child-environment events which *prevent* the development of motoric breakdown and ultimately, stuttering.

Preliminary descriptive information associated with a current clinical investigation (Proctor and Hanley, 1983) indicates that some children perceive changes of speech rate (syllables/minute), speech effort, or abrupt speech onset differently. For example, one child reliably identified changes of his mother's speech rate (video taped samples). Subsequent descriptions of that child's interactions with his mother (who again altered her speech rate) indicated that alterations of the child's speech rate approximated changes of his mother's speech rate, and increments of the child's rate were accompanied by increased disfluency. Another child was unable to reliably differentiate changes of his mother's speech rate (thus rate changes were not perceptually relevant for this child), and his speech rate remained stable when his mother spoke more rapidly during their subsequent interactions. A third child was similarly unable to detect his mother's increase of speech rate on video samples. His speech rate also remained relatively stable, even when his mother's rate of speech increased during their interactions. This child, however, became more disfluent when his mother spoke in an excited, forceful fashion (Mother was asked (a) to be "excited" and "forceful" during her interactions with her child and (b) maintain a speech rate which approximated her "habitual" level). The implications of these types of descriptions and observations are obvious. While we recognize that our observations may be at a rather superficial level which precludes knowledge of underlying events or mechanisms that contribute to disruption of coordination, such observations allow us to target events in the child's environment which are perceptually relevant to the child, and thus, may be very relevant clinically. The modification of a parent's speech rate may be relevant in one instance, whereas the modification of "effortful," "uncomfortable," or "excited" parent responses may be more important for other children or other speaking situations. By describing those "perceptual" events that are associated with breakdown of the child's speech and those associated with the child's fluent speech productions, we are in a better position to modify those events or conditions that are truly relevant. The following list suggests some of the possible conditions or behaviors which may be important as events which are environmentally relevant for certain children or in certain situations. As potentially relevant events, they may contribute to the child's processing of speech by serving as models, stimuli for reaction on the part of the child, or as cues regarding emotionality, level of expectation, etc., of other speakers.

SPEECH CHARACTERISTICS
OF FELLOW COMMUNICATORS
  • rate of speech (syllables/minute)
  • speed of movement (i.e., rapid, jerky movements of the articulators)
  • movement complexity (length of utterance, complex

movements associated with difficult phonemic combinations)
- stress or pitch variations related physiological adjustment
- speech characteristics of fellow speakers which are characterized by extreme tension, abrupt onset of voicing, etc.
- respiratory variations (rapid or abrupt respiratory patterns, truncated breath groups, inappropriate respiratory pauses)
- duration of phonemic, syllabic, or pausal segments
- speech patterns which are perceived as forceful, hesitant, cautious, or "over-controlled"

LINGUISTIC CHARACTERISTICS OF OTHER SPEAKERS IN THE CHILD'S ENVIRONMENT
- syntactic complexity
- vocabulary level of the speaker
- work retrieval strategies of the listener (pauses, interjections, revisions)
- morphological complexity of language structures
- length of utterance as a programmed unit of language

PSYCHOLOGICAL/EMOTIONAL FACTORS (How does the child perceive his listeners when exposed to their speech/language behavior?)
- excited
- comfortable
- hesitant
- withdrawn
- confident
- rushed
- supportive
- confused
- assertive
- patient
- aggressive
- panic ridden
- avoidant
- embarrassed

THE CHILD'S PERCEPTIONS OF OTHER SPEAKERS OR THE COMMUNICATIVE ENVIRONMENT WHICH CONVEY INFORMATION ABOUT THE SOCIAL INTERACTION TAKING PLACE
- behaviors which are perceived as extremely "authoritative" or "dominating"
- nonverbal/gestural behaviors of other speakers which are

perceived by the child as nervous or uncomfortable behaviors
- speech or nonverbal behaviors which are perceived by the child to reflect the listener's disinterest, reluctance, or critical judgemental affect

THE CHILD'S PERCEPTIONS OF THE COMMUNICATIVE SETTING OR NON-COMMUNICATIVE EVENTS WHICH OCCUR IN THAT SETTING

- noisy/distracting stimuli in the environment which may divert the child's attention or stimulate emotional reaction
- introduction of unfamiliar or novel objects, events, actions, or persons into the child's environments
- introduction of environmental events which minimize or enhance the child's visual awareness

This list is not inclusive, the categories are arbitrary, and the items listed may or may not be meaningful for each client. Only a careful description of the characteristics of each child, of different speaking situations, and of the child's perceptions of himself and those events in his environment will provide a list that is relevant for each case. The clinical activities used to gather such descriptions may vary (i.e., picture identification, spontaneous conversation, imitation, play therapy, etc.). The clinician should attempt to systematically alter communicative events which occur in the child's speaking environment(s) (i.e., emotionality, length of utterance, word stress patterns, syntactic complexity, etc.) to determine the effects of those alterations on the child's speech or nonverbal behavior. Those descriptions and manipulations will lead to the development of other activities that may be very helpful.

In keeping with the perspective described earlier, we recognize that perceptual phenomena and the events associated with them interact with other events classified as physiological, linguistic, psychological and environmental and that they should be considered in context with those events. The following section presents a brief review of speech motorics as they have been investigated and a discussion of those physiological events which may be relevant in light of the framework presented above.

The Study of Motor Processes in Children who Stutter

Our understanding of the motor processes which comprise normal speech production or stuttering is limited. The information pertaining to the motor processes of children, fluent or disfluent, is even more limited. Those investigations which have been completed have generally focused upon three areas related to motor performance: (1) The study of fine and gross motor performance of stuttering children, (2) The study of respiratory motor performance of stuttering children, (3) The study of acoustic phenomena (voicing, acoustic transitions produced during speech) which are related to speech motor processes. While the theme of each of these studies conveys an interest in motor control processes, most are obviously involved with measures at phenomenological levels (i.e., acoustic) which reflect events that emerge *from* motor processes. Such measures may be useful, but only if they have been related to other levels (movement, muscle, neural) of the speech production system. Until such relationships have been established, any conclusions drawn from such measures must be considered as speculative. Nonetheless, some of those investigations will be briefly described to provide the reader with an estimate of the limited information and understanding available regarding speech motorics of children who stutter. These investigations of *groups* of stutterers and *groups* of children with normal speech behavior are typical of other group investigations of stuttering phenomena in that they have yielded group findings which are inconclusive.

The study of gross and fine motor activities of children who stutter are reflected in the work of Westphal (1933), Cross (1936), Kopp (1946), and Finkelstein and Weisberger (1954). Westphal (1933) observed that twenty-six male, school-aged stutterers did not differ significantly when performance for motor tasks like bean bag tossing, or fitting pieces to a form board were attempted. Cross (1936) was unable to observe differences between stutterers and nonstutterers for a variety of motoric sorting and stacking tasks. Kopp (1946) used the Oseretsky test of motor performance to evaluate the motor behaviors of stuttering children (6½-15). Results suggested that stuttering children were somewhat retarded in motor development. A subsequent study of the performance of stuttering children on Oseretsky tasks (Finkelstein and Weisberger, 1954) contradicted Kopp's results. Stuttering children performed at an average of 7.3 months (motor age) above matched controls.

Some evidence of motor difficulty is presented in a series of studies which investigated the rhythmic abilities of children who stutter. Zaleski (1965) measured the rhythmic abilities of children (7-14) who stuttered by having them replicate a metronomic rhythm with tapping or repetitive speech gestures. Children who stuttered differed significantly more than nonstuttering children. Seth (1958) used a rapid tapping task as a test of motor rhythm for stuttering and control children. Left and right handed tapping patterns of stuttering children were inferior to normals. Martin (1962), however, was unable to observe any significant differences between stuttering and nonstuttering children for motor tasks which required rapid motor shifts in a mixture of fine motor tasks.

Murray (1932) analyzed thoracic pneumograms of stuttering and nonstuttering children as a measure of respiratory regularity or irregularity for normal breathing during silent reading, and during "reasoning" tasks. Stutterers had longer inspiration and expiration durations and were more variable on all measures. Steer (1935, 1937), in later respiratory studies observed that stuttering children did not evidence respiratory regularities which were different from nonstuttering children.

Stromsta (1965) measured the acoustic speech patterns of stuttering children. Acoustic characteristics were typefied by a lack of formant transitions and abrupt terminations of phonation. In a 10 year follow-up questionnaire, 24 of the original 27 stutterers who showed such irregularities were still stuttering. Ten of the 11 stutterers who originally showed normal transitions were reported to have stopped stuttering. Whether the measured differences reflect inherent motoric differences between stutterers or developmental motoric characteristics was not determined.

Recently, investigators have become very interested in the vocalization behavior of stuttering children. Wall, Starkweather, and Harris (1981) observed that stuttering in the speech of 4-6 year old children occurred more often on words which were initiated with voicing when they followed pause than when they were produced in running speech. Cullinan and Springer (1980) reported that children with stuttering as the only characteristic speech/language problem generally did not differ from nonstutterers in voice initiation time (duration between a stimulus tone and the onset of voicing for the production of "ah"). However, children who possessed speech and language problems in addition to stuttering were found to have significantly slower voice initiation times.

In two more recent studies, investigators made comparisons of voice reaction times and other motor behaviors (manual reaction times) in stuttering children. Cross and Luper (1983) reported that 5 and 9 year old stuttering children exhibited significantly longer and more variable voice and finger reaction times than did nonstutterers. Till, et. al. (1983), in contrast to Cross and Luper observed that stuttering children do not exhibit uniformly longer manual and phonatory reaction times than non-stuttering children.

Several theoretical or methodological issues may be generated from the consideration of the research findings described above. However, the following considerations seem reasonable as we develop or evaluate current clinical models:

1. The motor processes of young children who stutter may be *least* understandable if we consider their behavior in light of group data. Conflicting information and the high degree of variability observed within stuttering groups may suggest that individual stutterers are *not* members of a homogenous group of stutterers when measures such as those described above are considered.
2. The principles of operation of speech motor processes are not likely to be discovered if we continue to take measures at singular, discreet (i.e., behavior of the larynx) levels. Instead, the observation of patterns of behavior at various levels (emotional, muscle, neural, respiratory, laryngeal) may be more fruitful (Zimmermann, 1980).
3. Motorics may be best considered as an interactive component of a larger organismic-environmental system. The variability observed may be directly related to the interaction of the motor system to other organismic-environmental conditions.

Physiological Conditions

While the previous discussion reflects the need for researchers to experimentally measure relationships among different levels of the speech production system, clinicians should also recognize that assessments of such fluency disruptions as repetitions and prolongations reflect *our* perceptions of events which are clinically relevant indices of more fundamental physiological adjustments that have occurred at movement, muscle, neural, perceptual, or linguistic levels. We suspect that therapy procedures designed to shape or modify repetitions, prolongations, voice onsets, or airflow may be *effective* at times because they instigate changes at some other level of the speech production system (e.g., emotional inputs, background neural activity, speech rhythmicity, etc.). Such procedures may also be *ineffective* because they do not tap other levels or conditions necessary for normally fluent speech. This perspective suggests that therapy procedures should be "tailor made" to fit those unique conditions which have been described or associated with the child's stuttering problem. Children may do well with activities related to a certain level of speech production only if other conditions are also conducive to such adjustments. A given child may be successful if he/she is not extremely anxious, when using linguistic structures appropriate for the moment or situation, when they are confident, or when they perceive support and encouragement from their environment. Another child, in a different setting may benefit more readily from an adjustment of background muscle activity (i.e., through relaxation) or from modification of linguistic strategies. Again, the efficiency of the approach will vary for different children under different conditions. With this in mind we can carefully initiate our description of those physiological conditions that are hypothesized to be associated with disruptions.

At the acoustic level, we may perceive and describe pauses, repetitions, coarticulatory breakdown, etc. Those observations may lead us, by inference, to describe those movement or muscle adjustments that are related to discoordination. Our confidence in those inferences will depend on our understanding of the aerodynamic and mechanical principles of operation of the speech production system. For example, abnormal voice quality or abrupt onset of an acoustic speech signal should lead the clinician to suspect that muscles involved with the development of air pressures or laryngeal activity are not performing in a desirable fashion. In keeping with our frame of reference, those observed conditions may merely reflect adjustments of other (i.e., emotional, neural, perceptual) more elementary conditions associated with breakdown. Attempts to label the laryngeal maladjustments as responsible or "causal" may be erroneous or misleading. Such questionable implicit or explicit interpretations are often made by the reader of research on laryngeal behavior in stutterers. It is easy to become trapped into thinking that if the child has difficulty initiating voicing they have a defective "laryngeal system." The discussion above should indicate that this would be a very naive assumption. It is also unlikely that other observations such as the description of excessive lip tension during production of a plosive sound means that the lip, or the neural "wiring" going to the lip is faulty. It is more likely (given the lack of evidence to convince us otherwise) that inappropriate lip tension occurs because of some more central interaction of neural, reflexogenic, emotional, or linguistic events. Based upon current studies in movement control, Zimmermann, Smith, and

Hanley (1980) have hypothesized that such occurrences may result from changes of background neural activity, changes in triggering impulse, or both, and those changes may be sensitive to emotional or perceptual inputs.

A clinician was recently discussing the issues described above with her client, and she used a personal experience with her auto to convey to the client the danger of making premature or faulty assumption of "cause" when the principles of operation of a system (automobile or speech) are not completely understood:

An individual entered his auto, turned the key, and the engine started. The driver immediately noticed a "pinging" noise coming from the engine, a "coughing" noise coming from the exhaust pipe, and an engine noise which was definitely indicative of mistiming. Upon raising the hood for more careful observation, the driver noticed that the engine was noticeably vibrating and rocking on its mounts. He also noticed that the "pinging" noise came from the right front piston chamber of the engine. The driver looked no further. He immediately suspected that the noisy, "pingy" pistons were malfunctioning (and they were), and he decided that they would need to be replaced if he wanted his car to function normally. When the driver arrived at the service station to report the sad state of affairs to the auto mechanic, the mechanic undertook his own description of the problem. The driver was quite surprised when he saw the mechanic take a screwdriver from a box and gradually adjust a screw on the carburetor (which feeds gas to the engine) until the coughing, pinging, and rocking ceased. To the driver's surprise, the pistons were not defective. Rather, the input to the motor, which supplies energy (gasoline) to the engine was operating incorrectly.

This example makes one wonder how often the consumer has erred (often at considerable expense) in his premature diagnoses of mechanical problems. Similarly, the example should make one wonder how often clinicians or researchers have ignored important conditions associated with disfluency by pointing a "causal" finger at the child, the parent, the larynx, the air production system, etc. Until we completely understand the principles of operation of the speech production system (like the auto mechanic), we should be cautious with our interpretations of disrupted airflow, laryngeal blocks, or jerky speech movements. They may be indirect products of other more essential neurophysiological adjustments. In some cases, those observations may be only symptomatic phenomena which emerge from other, more essential interactions of events at other levels of the speech production system. For example a sympathetic "emotional" input into the brainstem networks may alter the pattern of neural activity which is *expressed* as laryngeal disfunction. In such a case, the emotional event may be a more significant variable than the laryngeal event.

Physiological Limits

Like any electromechanical system, the speech production system is subject to certain limitations. Muscles and speech structures operate most efficiently if they perform at optimal levels (force, tension, rate of movement, duration). The complexity of the movements generated by that system are also limited and unique for each individual. It should also be obvious that the limits of the system vary for different individuals at different developmental levels, for different sexes, and for different social, linguistic, and emotional states. In an experimental sense, then, we should be searching for an efficient therapy approach by systematically modifying those environmental (i.e., parent comments, number of listeners), linguistic (i.e., syntactic complexity, vocabulary, length of utterance, etc.), or listener behaviors which are perceived as uncomfortable, supportive, rushed, perfectionistic, etc. We should also observe psychosocial (i.e., communicative attitudes, self-percept, perception of listeners), or emotional (i.e., fears, feelings of panic, excitement) events to determine their relative effects on the child's threshold(s) or limits of discoordination or breakdown.

What modifications should be applied initially, and which conditions should receive the most emphasis in the clinic situation? The answer to that question must be discovered by the clinician. Those that have the most notable effect on fluency may be those that result in the most efficient modifications. However, brief attention given to those hypothesized to be less relevant often results in a pleasant clinical surprise. For example, an occasional "pep" talk with the young school age child about confidence or tenacity in the pursuit of fluency may provide a significant change in the child's performance in a number of communicative situations. For the preschool aged child, the clinician or parent's nonverbal cues of determination or confidence may accomplish the same purpose.

The measurement of frequency, intensity, and duration of

speech segments and the variation of these in clinic situations may help the child to alter or maintain physiological adjustments within threshold limits required for coordination. In some cases, however, those adjustments may be worthwhile in a limited number of settings, or only if emotional or linguistic conditions are compatable with those adjustments. For other situations, counseling regarding avoidance and fear, desensitization, relaxation, or modification of listener behavior may be more appropriate. The level of discussion must vary with the age and ability of the child. The preschooler will oftentimes relate best to nursery tales (i.e., *The Three Bears* for models of anger, *The Seven Dwarfs* for models of relaxation, or *Little Red Riding Hood* for a portrayal of disguise or fear).

Clinicians may often ignore some of their perceptual evaluations or descriptors of the child's communicative behavior because they have been taught to think that there is little clinical relevance in events which cannot be easily measured or do not fit into traditional categories of speech rate, phoneme duration, voice onset time, etc. This may not only be a faulty assumption, but it may lead us to place false confidence in variables that are less relatable to physiological processes than some of our less "objective" intuitions and feelings.

If the clinician perceives that the child is extremely "careful," "hesitant," or "hurried," the physiological adjustments which underlie the "careful" or "hesitant" behaviors may be significantly related to the promotion of speech breakdown. They may reflect alterations of physiological force, the development of aberrant "emotional" inputs to the motor system, inappropriate neurolinguistic activity, etc. Any of these adjustments may place the speech production system in an unstable mode which enhances the likelihood of malfunction. The child who is normally fluent but extremely "hesitant" or "cautious" while speaking may be operating very close to a threshold for breakdown. Such "at risk" modes may be akin to the coordination difficulties experienced by the adult who attempts to learn to drive an automobile in a very cautious, "over-controlled" fashion, or to the child who "carefully" attempts to walk on a balance beam. When we observe speech modes or "strategies" such as those described, we have just reason to pursue clinical activities which promote "less effortful" (i.e., more relaxed), less "rapid," or less cautious ("free and easy") speech modes. There is even reason to suspect that these types of general alterations may be for some circumstances more efficient modification goals than therapy activities which focus upon a particular muscular set or articulator structure because they may be more closely related to adjustments which most efficiently "stabilize" the speech production system. A discussion of control and co-ordination of movement by Kelso, Tuller, and Harris (1983) is related to this topic.

The clinician should also be aware of the possible inefficiency and risk of error of description or interpretation that may result when we impose our own vocabularies and "causal" presuppositions on our observations (i.e., behaviors or events described as "conditioned negative emotions," "operants," or "objective attitudes"). The use of these and similar vocabularies increase rather than decrease the likelihood of bias and lack of objectivity in our clinician activity. We should similarly recognize that a primary communicative barrier to effective client/clinician/parent interaction involves the use of irrelevant vocabulary. Children often relate more readily to events which characterize their speech performance, communicative strategies, or perceptual experiences when they attach their own (often unique) vocabularies to the conditions described. A child's reports of "letting it all hang out," "letting it all go," or "backing off" represent the child's interpretation (at some related level) of physiological adjustments that are conducive to fluent speech. Those vocabularies may be more related to "significant" adjustments than *imposed* clinician vocabularies connoting releasing, freezing, relaxing, reprogramming, cancelling, etc. If a child expresses caution or hesitancy with statements such as "walking on eggshells," "tiptoeing through the tulips," or "walking a tightrope," those evaluations may be closely related to the actual neural adjustments which have taken place. Recently, a young child enamoured by automobiles made reference to his speech with metaphoric descriptions which were relevant for him. His description of "peeling out from a stop sign" (possibly to denote a hurried, abrupt movement), "attempting to drive a Volkswagon like a Camaro" (i.e., over-exerting, excessively forcing, or stressing the speech system), "flooding the engine" (i.e., harsh, abrupt onset of speech energy, and overflow of such), and "over-steering" (to depict his efforts to over-control his speech movements) proved to be very meaningful clinician constructs, and the activities designed around them were quite meaningful and efficient.

The clinical techniques that might be used to address various physiological and perceptual conditions which have been identified are numerous, and they must be discovered by the clinician. Clinical techniques that involve shaping of more desirable behaviors, counseling regarding inappropriate perceptions and emotional reactions, modeling/imitation, role adjustment, and others may contain elements that are useful. We should also make comparisons of the efficiency of our various procedures aimed directly at the speech movements or movement dysfunction (i.e., attempts to directly modify lip tension, voice onset, or airflow) to those procedures (i.e., relaxation, getting set to initiate "easily," "starting in" smoothly, etc.) which *may* tap adjustments at other more fundamental levels (i.e., background neural level) in a more efficient manner.

Linguistic Considerations

Each child possesses a linguistic capability based upon genetic factors and experience. The neural events associated with language processing are constantly interacting, at some unknown levels, with other physiological, emotional, psychological, and environmental events. Just as the child's speech motor capability is subject to some limits of performance and some optimal level of performance, so is his linguistic potential. Linguistic conditions, then interact with some other communicative events to enhance or disrupt fluent speech production. The "limits" of those linguistic conditions may differ at different ages of development, with changes of emotionality, or in different settings. As is true of many other aspects of the human communication system, the linguistic "processes" are still quite mysterious. However, we can be quite confident that a child's ability to process language and to formulate his "expressive" language efficiently and competently will contribute to linguistic "conditions" of fluency or disfluency. Careful description of the child's syntactical structures, morphological forms, vocabulary, length of utterance, and the pragmatic aspects of his language may elucidate relevant linguistic events or conditions which require clinical attention.

Just as our measures of excessive rate, speech effort, hesitancy, etc., may reflect significant physiological breakdown, the word revisions noted in a child's speech as he searches for a more appropriate syntactical form may exemplify the interactions between linguistic and psychological processes. Similarly, we can recognize that our difficulty selecting appropriate expressive vocabulary when we are standing in front of a classroom full of students may represent an interaction of emotional and linguistic events, and the physiological adjustments which result (tense speech movements, blotching, sweating, averted eye movement, etc.) are probably unique to that specific interaction. These linguistic conditions may not be immediately apparent if we rely on "normative" measures taken from formal tests or from the language development literature. For.example, one child may be evaluated (on a formal syntax screening test) to have a syntactical problem. However, his rank, or score, may have little or nothing to do (as a significant condition) with the fluency of his speech. He may go through life being syntactically inappropriate, but very fluent. Another child may score above the norm on the same test. However, if he chooses to implement syntactical structures which are beyond his limits, he may invoke a condition (syntactic, linguistic) that is conducive, by interaction with other events, to the breakdown of speech motor processes. Enhancement of the second child's syntactical ability (even though it is above normal performance to begin with) may represent a "significant" alteration of a condition associated with the establishment of fluency. Similarly, a parent language model which is very complex syntactically may be an important condition for the child with restricted syntactical abilities, but unimportant for a child who is proficient syntactically. The only way we can determine the relevance of a "syntactical" condition of disfluency for the second child is by carefully describing and estimating his basic syntactical abilities, estimating his syntactical structures in various settings, and using the observed discrepancies to hypothesize that a significant "syntactical" condition may exist. From the example provided above, we can suspect that an alternative clinical procedure (i.e., counseling or modeling) will help the child adjust his expressive language "back to" normal limits. Similar descriptions and comparisons may be made for other linguistic variables to estimate the child's best limits, the limits of his current performance, the discrepancy which exists, and alternative approaches to be tested. Again such descriptions and comparisons must take place with careful notation of other physiological (i.e., speech rate, effort), emotional (i.e., level of "excitement"), or environmental (i.e., parent behaviors or reactions) events which are contextually associated to and interactive with the child's linguistic capability or performance.

Psychosocial Considerations

As part of our clinical description and the procedures we develop during our work with the child, we should carefully estimate and describe those psychosocial variables (communicative personality, psychological "sets," communicative or situational fears, nonverbal behavior, perceived affect, etc.) which may interact with other conditions during the communication process. Certain "personality" traits or "communicative themes" will often characterize conversation about certain topics, interaction with certain individuals or types of individuals, or certain environmental settings. The child who is judged to be "atypically" disfluent may not only be experiencing difficulty with speech coordination, but he may also experience difficulty because his communicative style, his level of conversation, or his linguistic structures are not acceptable (to him and/or to his listener) for a given situation or experience. Again, it should be obvious that events related to social type, affect, etc., will interact with listener variables or with other linguistic or emotional conditions to promote aberrant physiological adjustment. The client's reported feelings of being "helpless," feelings of "panic," "insecurity," "frustration," etc., may be reflections of perceptions which are associated with an emotional reaction to a discoordinated speech activity in a social situation. Rather than using the "chicken and the egg" method of questioning (i.e., Did the emotion cause the discoordination? Did the discoordination cause the listener to react? Was an aversive stimulus present in the environment which acted as a "punisher" of coordinated speech movement?), which will probably lead nowhere, we might more appropriately hypothesize that each of these conditions (social listener, emotionality, and discoordination) were part of a "unitary" communicative process. They represent interactions. They represent events which characterize a communicative or ecological set of circumstances. To consider them as discreet variables, or to fit them into categories of "stimulus" and "response" or "cause" and "effect" may be an inaccurate characterization of their import. If we describe them as associated psychosocial events which, through perceptual or sensory channels, are interfaced with the motor neuron system, we can hypothesize that they are "significant" or important conditions of breakdown. More "sophisticated" interpretations are not yet defendable, at least in terms of vocabulary which allows them to be tested.

A child who is describing his recent experiences at the circus may begin to describe his experiences in a very "excited" fashion. With his eyes wide open, he may begin his description with an abrupt, deep inhalation, a forceful onset of voicing followed by an endless sentence spoken at a very rapid rate of speech. As we observe a tense sound repetition at the beginning of the sentence (I-I-I-I-I went . . .), should we assume that the adductory muscles of the larynx are malfunctioning (surely they are), or should we assume that rapid speech rate is the culprit? Does his extreme emotionality cause those repetitions, or is it because his utterances are too long? Maybe his mother isn't being a good listener??? All of those factors may be involved in some way, and the interaction of all of them probably effect aberrant physiological adjustments. It is possible that the clinician or child may be able to modify any one of those variables to develop more fluent speech patterns. Possibly, several need to be altered to promote fluent behavior. Alteration of *the* event (or combination of events) which is most efficient or meaningful must be determined by tests of clinical hypotheses. Listener events which are perceptually relevant for the child, linguistic structures, emotionality, and processes of coordination must all be considered as part of the recipe.

Conclusion

This discussion was not intended to address the question "What should I do with the child who stutters? It is assumed that the clinician already possesses the basic skills to counsel, describe, measure, and implement modification procedures. Instead, this discussion was intended to present a perspective (which may already be obvious to many) which promotes the consideration of the child as a communicating, interacting individual who possess those motoric disruptions we often label as stuttering. It was suggested that if we consider events at a number of different levels (physiological, psychological, social, linguistic, emotional, etc.) which may interact to promote maladjustments of the physiological underpinnings of disfluency, we may be able to discover (by experimentation in the clinic or home setting) a most efficient set of procedures for that child. By careful description of all events which we consider to be potentially relevant, we can only hope that we might discover the procedures which will benefit each child who, by his unique characteristics and communicative experiences, will contribute to the human experience in a positive, happy manner.

References

Cross, D., and Luper, H., "The Relation Between Finger Reaction Time and Voice Reaction Time in Stuttering and Nonstuttering Children and Adults," *Journal of Speech and Hearing Research*, 26, 356-361, 1983.

Cross, H. M., "The Motor Capacities of Stutterers," *Archives of Speech*, 1, 112-132, 1936.

Cullinan, W. L., and Springer, M. T., "Voice Initiation and Termination Times in Stuttering and Nonstuttering Children," *Journal of Speech and Hearing Research*, 23, 344-360, 1980.

Finkelstein, P., and Weisberger, S., "The Motor Proficiency of Stutterers," *Journal of Speech and Hearing Disorders*, 19, 52-59, 1954.

Johnston, J., and Turvey, M. T., "A Sketch of an Ecological Metatheory for Theories of Learning," in Bower, G. H. (Ed.), *The Psychology of Learning and Motivation*. New York: Academic Press, 1980.

Johnson, W., and Associates, *The Onset of Stuttering*. Minneapolis: University of Minnesota Press, Chapter 10, 1959.

Kelso, J. A. Scott, Tuller, B., and Harris, K., "A 'Dynamic Pattern' Perspective on the Control of Coordination in Movement," in MacNeilage, P. (Ed.), *The Production of Speech*. New York: Springer-Verlag, 137-166, 1983.

Kopp, H., "Psychosomatic Study of Fifty Stuttering Children: II Oseretsky Tests," *American Journal of Orthopsychiatry*, 16, 114-119, 1946.

Martin, R. R., "Stuttering and Perseveration in Children," *Journal of Speech and Hearing Research*, 5 332-339, 1962.

Murray, E., "Disintegration of Breathing and Eye Movements in Stuttering During Silent Reading and Reasoning," *Psychological Monographs*, 43, 218-275, 1932.

Proctor, L., and Hanley, J., *Effort, Rate, and Rhythmicity: Perception-production Perspectives in Stuttering*. Presented at the American Speech and Hearing Association National Convention, Cincinnati, November, 1983.

Shettlesworth, S., "Function and Mechanism in Learning," in Zeilerang, M., and Harzem, P. (Eds.), *Advances in Analysis of Behavior. Volume 3: Biological Factors in Learning*. New York: Wiley and Sons, 1982.

Steer, M. D., "A Qualitative Study of Breathing in Young Stutterers," *Speech Monographs*, 2, 152-156, 1935.

Stromsta, C., "A Spectrographic Study of Dysfluencies Labeled as Stuttering By Parents," *Ed Therapia Vocis et Loquelae*, 1, XIII, Congress of The International Society of Logopedics and Phoniatrics, 317-320, 1965.

Till, J., Reich, A., Dickey, S., and Sieber, J., "Phonatory and Manual Reaction Times of Stuttering and Nonstuttering Children, *Journal of Speech and Hearing Research*, 26, 171-181, 1983.

VanRiper, C., *The Nature of Stuttering (Second Ed.)*. Englewood Cliffs, New Jersey: Prentice-Hall, 1982.

Wall, M., Starkweather, C. W., and Harris, K., "The Influence of Voicing Adjustment on the Location of Stuttering in the Spontaneous Speech of Young Stutterers," *Journal Fluency Disorders*, 6, 299-311, 1981.

Westphal, G., "An Experimental Study of Certain Motor Abilities of Stutterers," *Child Development*, 4, 214-221, 1933.

Zaleski, T., "Rhythmic Skills in Stuttering Children," *Ed Therapia Vocis et Loquelae*, 1, 37-41, 1965.

Zimmermann, G., "Stuttering: A Disorder of Movement," *Journal of Speech and Hearing Research*, 23, 122-136, 1980.

Zimmermann, G., and Hanley, J., *A Perception-production Approach to Stuttering*. Presentation to the North Central Regional Conference of ASHA, Milwaukee, August, 1982.

Zimmermann, G., and Kelso, J. Scott, "Remarks on the 'Causal' Basis of Stuttering," to be Published in the *Proceeding of the VanRiper Lecture Series*, Kalamazoo, Michigan, April, 1982.

Zimmermann, G., Smith, A., and Hanley, J., "Stuttering: In Need of a Unifying Conceptual Framework," *Journal of Speech and Hearing Research*, 24, 25-31, 1981.

chapter four

The Development of Fluency in Normal Children

C. Woodruff Starkweather, Ph.D.
Temple University

I. Introduction

The Concept of Fluency

The word fluency means flowing along. It was used originally to refer to the way a person spoke a second language. If the language could be produced easily, smoothly, and quickly then the person was fluent in the language. Stutterers are described as not being fluent, although the word clearly means something else in this use because it has always been recognized that, unlike the person who is not fluent in a second language, a stutterer, at least a confirmed or adult stutterer, knows what to say and how to pronounce it but is just unable to produce it easily or quickly. This suggests that we need to distinguish between speech fluency and language fluency.

Second-language learners are fluent if they can easily and quickly encode their intentions into the conventional form. They lack language fluency if they cannot easily or quickly find the right words (semantically nonfluent), pronounce them (phonologically nonfluent), arrange them in order (syntactically nonfluent), or use them appropriately for the circumstances (pragmatically nonfluent). Uncertainty and nonfluency are closely related. The word "fluent," when referring to second language skill, may connote superiority, whereas it connotes normality in referring to first language, speech production skill. Fillmore (1979) has described three types of superior speakers as fluent in different ways corresponding roughly to semantic, syntactic, and pragmatic fluency. The semantically fluent individual has a large vocabulary and ready access to it for referral to many different concepts. The syntactically fluent speaker can encode sentences of great complexity to represent ideas that are equally complex in their internal relations. The pragmatically fluent speaker always knows how to say the right thing under many different circumstances. Fillmore did not describe phonological fluency, but we would guess that phonologically fluent speakers find it easy to pronounce long and difficult words and phrases.

In most cases, these are not the skills that confirmed or adult stutterers lack as part of their disorder. One can be a severe stutterer and yet still have (a) a large and useful vocabulary, (b) the ability to compose complex sentences, (c) the knowledge of what sentences are appropriate for the communication of a given intention under specific circumstances, and (d) the knowledge of how words are pronounced. So one can stutter and still be linguistically fluent. What the adult or confirmed stutterer lacks is speech fluency. However, there are some close relations between speech and language fluency which make it difficult at times to distinguish them. Also, in children patterns of growth and development may influence both language and speech fluency and create a closer relationship between the two types of behavior in children more than in adults. To look at the relation between speech and language fluency in children, Kline and Starkweather (1977) gathered 100-utterance samples of the spontaneous speech of 4-6 year old stutterers in their homes. The Test for the Auditory Comprehension of Language (TACL) (Carrow, 1973) short form was given to each of the children. Then, a very closely matched sample of nonstutterers — matched for age within 3 months, for sex, for classroom, socioeconomic level, and general achievement — was identified. The language samples were segmented and analyzed for Mean Length of Utterance (MLU). The stutterers produced significantly shorter utterances and significantly lower TACL scores than the nonstutterers. Also, their TACL scores were positively correlated with their MLU. We concluded that the stutterers were a little slow in acquiring language skills, and it seemed unlikely (although not impossible) that this lag was secondary to the stuttering, since it showed up in a comprehension test as well.

Let us look now at the concept of speech fluency. Wendell Johnson (1956; 1961) had a major impact on our thinking about stuttering and fluency. He believed that stuttering developed from the way others reacted to young speakers' hesitations and repetitions, and he made a point of explaining that it was really quite normal for young children to stumble often in their speech. These "nonfluencies" were seen as "normal." Although most children seem to stop repeating sounds as they get older, it is important to recognize several important facts. First, there are different types of nonfluencies in children, as in adults, and they follow different courses of development. One type in particular — frequent and long part-word repetitions — seem to appear spontaneously in some (but not all) children. Most parents react to the occurrence of this type of nonfluency by saying that their child is stuttering. Many speech and language clinicians too are coming to call this pattern of nonfluency stuttering. Although as many as 75-80 percent of stutterers may recover spontaneously (Sheehan and Martyn, 1970), the remaining 20-25 percent begin to struggle and force and end up stuttering. So it is at least questionable whether this particular type of behavior is "normal." It might be better to use a word like "benign" or call them "developmental disfluencies," as some writers have done. The problem with these terms is the remaining 20-25 percent who become stutterers. For these children, disfluencies turn out not to be a benign developmental phase.

Johnson believed that those children whose parents overreacted to these disfluencies became stutterers. So it was important for him to emphasize the normality of this behavior. As a result of Johnson's emphasis, we have been much concerned with normal nonfluencies. We have been relatively unconcerned about the development of normal fluency except with regard to the continuity of young children's speech. Speech/language clinicians are trained to evaluate articulation disorders against a background of language development. But in the area of fluency, most clinicians evaluate stuttering only by counting the frequency of disfluent words and by observing qualitative characteristics, including the amount of struggle that is present. Our evaluations of young stutterers would be improved by considering fluency more broadly, by looking at the rate, the rhythm, and the ease with which children speak, as well as the continuity of their speech. As children mature they become increasingly proficient at producing speech sounds, and this growing proficiency is seen in a faster rate of syllable production, briefer pauses, and more extensive coarticulation of adjacent sounds. The frequency with which disfluencies occur, on the other hand, does not show such a clear developmental pattern. Some types of disfluencies become less frequent, others do not change, and a few increase in frequency as children grow. Because fluency seems to be more than the continuity of speech production, I prefer to use the word "discontinuity" to label pauses, hesitations, whole and part-word repetitions and other breaks in the forward flow of speech instead of the word "disfluency." "Discontinuity" seems more precise than "disfluency."

In another paper (Starkweather, 1980), I tried to identify the different measures one could make of speech fluency. I was interested in determining what varied with speech fluency and how it changed as children developed. In reviewing the literature, it became apparent that fluency consisted of more than just the absence of nonfluencies, but that, in addition fluent speech was rapid and effortless. So it seemed to me that there were three basic dimensions to speech fluency: (1) the rate of speech, (2) the continuity of speech, and (3) the effort or ease with which speech is produced. As it turned out, these "dimensions," were inter-related. They were correlated with each other and with another variable — information load or uncertainty. More recently, I have come to believe that effort, or the ease with which sounds can be produced, is more central to the theoretical concept of fluency, than rate or continuity. It is tempting to suggest that fluency *is* ease of speech, and that continuity and rate are observable results of it.

It will be useful now to consider each aspect of normal speech fluency in more detail. An attempt will be made to determine empirical bases for the clinical evaluation of fluency. Be warned, however, that the empirical bases will be hard to find. Our lack of interest in normal fluency has led to a small research effort.

II. The Development of Continuity

Yairi (1981) has conducted the only longitudinal study of speech continuity in normal children. He observed normally speaking two-year-old boys and girls three times during the course of a year at four month intervals. Samples of spontaneous speech, 500 words long, were obtained at each observation. There was extreme diversity in the data, some children showing virtually no discontinuities, while the two most disfluent children produced 13 and 25 discontinuities per 100 words spoken. There was no difference between the sexes, although there were more boys in the "highly disfluent" category. During the year, there were sharp fluctuations in the frequency of discontinuities. The older children (32-40 months) showed a decline. The younger children (25-37 months) showed an increase. This latter group was observed at an additional four month interval, at which time the beginning of a decline was apparent. These trends, however, were observed against a background of diversity, and Yairi concluded that the continuity of speech did not follow a predictable developmental course in two-year-olds.

There have also been a few stratified studies. Haynes and Hood (1977) observed 30 nonstuttering children ages 4, 6, and 8. Fifty utterances (complete sentence) were obtained. They did not find significant differences in the frequency of discontinuities by age or sex, although there was an increase in the number of interjections between ages 4 and 8. More recently, Wexler and Mysak (1982) have observed the discontinuities of 36 nonstuttering males aged 2, 4, and 6. They found no change in the distribution of fluency types at the different ages. However, they did find that the youngest group produced a higher frequency of discontinuity than the two older groups. They also found that certain types of discontinuities were related to certain other types, specifically revision-incomplete phrase, interjections, and whole word repetitions seemed to be related, and they considered these "linguistically based disfluencies," while part-word repetitions and disrhythmic phonations formed a second group, which they considered "motorically based."

In none of these studies, however, was any aspect of fluency other than discontinuity observed. There has been only one study (Kowal, O'Connell, and Sabin, 1975) in which discontinuities have been observed along with other aspects of fluency, such as rate and pause duration. Kowal, O'Connell and Sabin asked 12 boys and 12 girls at each of 7 age groups from kindergarten through high school seniors to describe a series of Snoopy cartoons. Afterwards, the recordings were analyzed for the number of syllables spoken, the number and type of discontinuities, the rate of speech in syllables per second, the number of syllables per unfilled pause, and the duration of unfilled pauses per syllable. The results of this study are particularly relevant to this discussion because the analysis was more comprehensive and because they provide data for the school-aged child, with whom most clinical work is done. They supplement the work discussed earlier on the preschool child. Diagnosis is typically made before the child enters school, but evaluation and the setting of clinical goals continue into the school years in many cases. Consequent-

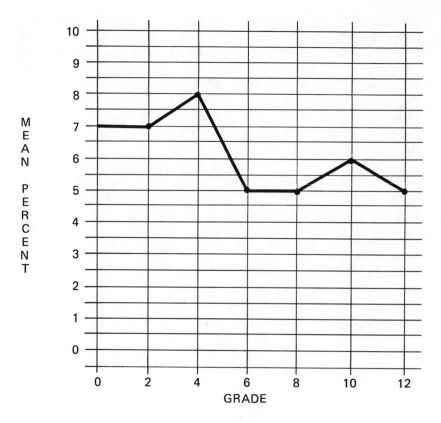

FIGURE 1
The Mean Frequency of All Discontinuities by Grade Level

ly, the results of this study will be presented in considerable detail. Figure 1 shows the mean percentage of "vocal hesitations" per syllable for each of the seven age groups. "Vocal hesitations" consisted in this study of filled pauses (um, uh, hm), false starts, repeated words or parts of words, and parenthetical remarks. It is clear that there is very little change in the total frequency of discontinuities from kindergarten through high school. There is a small downward trend, but it is no more than two percent. The number of discontinuities per syllable does not seem to be an aspect of normal speech fluency that shows very much development after the preschool years. This is consistent with other observations of the discontinuities of school-aged children (Wexler and Mysak, 1982; Haynes and Hood, 1977), but it still seems odd because other measures, which we will come to shortly, do show development during this period.

As we shall see, there are problems involved in using frequency of discontinuities as a measure of fluency. For one, there are several different types of discontinuities, and developmental effects are masked when all discontinuities are lumped together as a single category. Figures 2 and 3 show the number of discontinuities per thousand syllables for individual types of discontinuities. Filled pauses per thousand syllables are shown in Figure 2. A modest decline can be seen. In absolute terms, the frequency of filled pauses only declines a few per thousand during 12 years of development. Figure 2 also shows the frequency of false starts. In this case there is a noticeable decline, to about a third of their level in kindergarten. Figure 3 shows

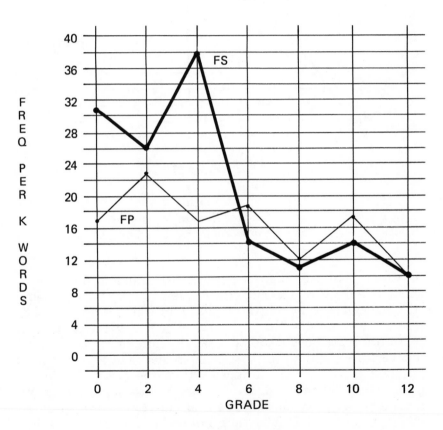

FIGURE 2
*The Frequency of False Starts
and Filled Pauses by Grade Level*

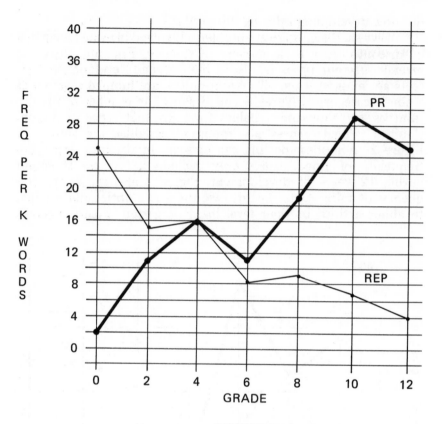

FIGURE 3
The Frequency of Repetitions
and Parenthetical Remarks by Grade Level

repetitions and parenthetical remarks. The repetitions decline to about one sixth of the kindergarten level by senior year. Note that the category of repetitions includes whole-word as well as part-word repetitions. Kowal, O'Connell, and Sabin observed that part-word repetitions made up a sizeable proportion of the total number of repetitions in the kindergarteners and second-graders but that it had all but dropped out of the picture by fourth grade. With this in mind, the increase in false starts and repetitions that occurs at fourth grade is an interesting reversal of the developmental trend. It is more noticeable for false starts than for repetitions. I would simply guess that it is at about this time in development when children may begin trying to talk more "correctly," under the influence of the formal teaching of grammar for purposes of written composition. As they try to "edit" their speech, they become more hesitant and correct themselves more often.

The developmental trend for the frequency of parenthetical remarks is different from that for the other types. While the frequency of filled pauses remains stable and false starts and repetitions decline, the frequency of parenthetical remarks increases from only two per thousand syllables in kindergarten to 25 per thousand syllables in senior year. These data are consistent with those of Haynes and Hood (1977) who found an increase in the number of interjections and a decrease in the number of whole word repetitions. All of the researchers observed a sharply higher variability in the youngest age groups.

It seems fair to describe these data as showing that kindergarteners' speech is not much less continuous than high school seniors', but the occurrence of some *forms* of discontinuity at older ages are representative of immaturity. False starts are somewhat immature, repetitions are quite immature, and part-word repetitions are very immature. In addition, part-word repetitions show a correspondence with other measures of fluency, which, as we shall see, these other types of discontinuities lack. With development, these immature types of discontinuities are replaced with more sophisticated types, of which the parenthetical remark — "well," "you know," "I mean" — is typical. In very well educated adults, the disfluencies may get even more sophisticated. Unfortunately, Kowal, O'Connell, and Sabin did not report standard deviations in this part of their study, so it is not possible to say how much an individual child should deviate from these means before being considered deviant. A number of studies were done in the thirties and forties on the disfluencies of preschool children by age, but these also did not report the standard deviations for different types of disfluencies. Davis (1939), in her study of preschool children aged two to five, found that repetitions occurred at a mean frequency of 49 per thousand for the group as a whole, which seems about right, when compared to Kowal, O'Connell, and Sabin's data for older children. Yairi (1981) reported means and standard deviations for the two-year-olds in his study but found the data so variable that he concluded that means were not an adequate representation of central tendency. One research need, clearly, is a large sample study of fluency, including continuity, rate, stress patterns, and the durations of speech sounds and pauses in preschool children.

The Nature of Disfluencies

It will be useful to take a closer look at the kind of behavior involved in these discontinuities. Are they slips and stumbles in the forward flow of speech, that is, are they really momentary disruptions of fluency, or do they serve some purpose? It seems "what I mean to say" is more than a stumble. It stalls for time, lets us keep talking, while we think or plan or edit. It may not have very much meaning — indeed its purpose is to fill up time at a point when the speaker has nothing meaningful ready to produce — but it is too coordinated and studied a use of language to be considered a stumble. The parenthetical remark appears to be just a more elaborate version of the filled pause. It is a way of keeping the floor while giving the speaker a little more time to produce the next utterance. Seen in this way, the filled pause and the parenthetical remark are certainly not errors. In fact they are rather more like corrections than errors, at least they provide the time for corrections of thought or of language to occur before utterance. The language that parenthetical remarks are composed of suggests this purpose, even though they are used without much regard for their meaning. "Do you know what I mean?" "Understand?" "I mean, I mean." If we can accept the idea that parenthetical remarks serve a correcting function by providing speakers with time to revise or better plan their utterance, it should not be difficult to see the false start also as a kind of correction, really the same kind of correction, except that the error wasn't quite detected before utterance began. A speaker begins to say something, gets part way into it and then realizes that it would lead to an ungrammatical sentence, an incongruous thought, an illogical conclusion, an indefensible position, be socially inappropriate, lead to a word of uncertain meaning, or any number of "mistakes." Before going any farther, the speaker stops and starts over again on a better course. Surely, that can be seen as a correction, not an error. Even in the case of repetitions, it may be that when young children repeat a whole word or a phrase they are stalling for time in just the same way older children do by saying "uh" or "Ya knowwaddimean." So all of the discontinuities that are vocalized, with the important exception of the part-word repetition, seem to be corrections, or serve a correcting function. They seem not to be stumbles, slips, or errors in the production of speech. These discontinuities, incidentally, also help the listener in a number of different ways. They are conversational devices (Starkweather, 1980).

The odd thing about these discontinuities is the persistent

belief that people seem to have that they are errors of speech. Of course, there are superior speakers who have very few of these discontinuities — highly fluent, they never need to stall for time or correct themselves because they get it right the first time.

It may be deleterious for children to be told to "correct" these corrections. They may try to talk faster so as to rush by them, or push hard to get the words out, or just get very tense muscularly as they try to make their speech mechanisms do something they are not equipped to do. These misguided attempts at "correction" may even lead to other behaviors that are even less desirable, and which may require further correction, and so on, down a very rapid spiral to a point from which extrication is not easy. This may be one way tense and struggled disfluency develops.

Clinical Applications

It is possible to derive, from the data we have seen here, some guidelines to use in evaluating individual children in the clinic. It should be recognized that the appropriate procedure for making clinical decisions about individual clients is to compare the client with standardized norms. We do not have such norms. Instead, we have a limited sample, adequate for research purposes, but not large enough or representative enough to be a standard. But the clinical imperative is strong. We hope these guidelines will be revised as genuine standardized norms are achieved. They have been prepared by smoothing the curves presented earlier, by connecting the midpoints of adjacent segments, and then interpolating for the missing grades, again by using the midpoints of adjacent segments. The curves were smoothed because with such a small sample, a portion of the fluctuations in the curve is probably attributable to sampling error. The result is a table of profiles for the different types of discontinuities at different grade levels (Table I).

Since there are no standard deviations provided for discontinuities in Kowal, O'Connell, and Sabin's data, and since it appears that we are dealing with a developing ability, we can report deviations from the norm in terms of grade level. For example, a child in the third grade who produces 14 parenthetical remarks per thousand syllables is at the fifth or sixth grade level. Preschool continuity is simply too variable to speculate about. It is important to distinguish between part-word and whole-word or phrase repetitions. Kowal, O'Connell, and Sabin tell us only that 24 per cent of the total number of repetitions for all ages were part-word repetitions, and these were distributed

TABLE I
Discontinuity Profiles for Schoolchildren

	Mean Frequency per 1,000 Syllables				
Grade	Filled Pauses	False Starts	Repetitions	Parenthetical Remarks	Totals
K	18	29	23	4	73
1	19	28	20	7	74
2	20	27	18	10	74
3	19	26	16	12	73
4	19	26	14	14	72
5	18	22	12	14	65
6	17	18	10	14	59
7	17	15	9	17	57
8	17	12	8	20	55
9	16	12	8	23	57
10	16	12	7	26	59
11	14	11	6	26	56
12	13	11	5	26	54

among the younger children, from kindergarten to fourth grade.

The continuity of speech is also broken up by silent or unfilled pauses. These tend to be shorter than pauses that are filled but not so short as juncture pauses. At one time it was felt that the two different types of pauses reflected different processes because they were distributed in the language differently. Specifically, the filled pauses were likely to occur at clause boundaries and before content words, while the unfilled pauses occurred more often before function words and within clauses. It seems now, however, as if the important difference between the two types of pauses is their length, the longer pauses reflecting syntactic locations of greater uncertainty. When the uncertainty is very high, as at a clause boundary, the pause is very long, and when it gets beyond a certain length, it is filled by the speaker so as to retain the floor. The syntactic structure of the utterance also predisposes the listener to expect that there might be a change or turn at a clause boundary. Consequently, it is a little more important to fill pauses at these locations, if you want to keep on talking. Kowal, O'Connell, and Sabin (1975) did not count the frequency of unfilled pauses. They saw these pauses as indicators of syntactic planning and, since they were interested in the psycholinguistic implications of their data, they measured the duration of unfilled pauses. Consequently, it will be more convenient for us to consider this type of pause in the next section.

III. The Development of Rate

The relationship of pauses to rate requires discussion. Of course, the pause takes up time and consequently slows down the rate of speech. This is, in a way, the listener's point of view, but the speaker is more active during pauses and sees it from a different point of view. For the speaker, the rate of speech may be said to vary continuously. When it slows down a great deal and comes to a halt, that is a pause. As the pause lengthens, the rate of speech may be considered as taking negative values. This is a handy way to conceptualize rate so as to allow the continuous variable rate to coexist happily with the discrete variable continuity.

The rate of speech, as indicated by the duration of segments, speeds up after a pause and then gradually slows down until the next pause (Umeda, 1975; 1977). This suggests that pauses may help speakers produce speech rapidly by giving them a chance to prepare for a sequence of gestures. It is the same reason a football team huddles before each play — to make sure all the parts function together and the timing is right to execute the sequence of events without error. What is curious about this is that if pauses help to achieve a more rapid rate, i.e., if they gain more time than they lose, and if rate is a part of speech fluency, then pauses help to achieve fluency. The frequency with which they occur would not then be a good measure of fluency, since the occurrence of a pause may promote fluency. But we have been calling them disfluencies. How can disfluencies work *for* fluency? The problem is in using the word "disfluency" to describe pauses. It is only when pauses are abnormally long or filled in ways that reflect immature fluency that they are "disfluent." So, the duration, but not the frequency, of pauses seems to reflect fluency.

It will be useful now to discuss Kowal, O'Connell, and Sabin's (1975) findings with regard to the duration of unfilled pauses. They defined unfilled pauses as any silence longer than 270 msec.

As a result, some of the longer juncture pauses were probably included in their data. Since they were thinking of the length of the unfilled pause as a measure of language planning, they divided the length of each unfilled pause by the number of syllables in the subsequent utterance. Their results can be seen in Figure 4. It is clear that the length of unfilled pauses shows a

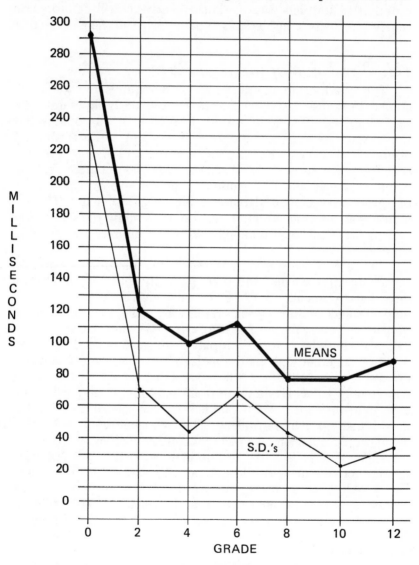

FIGURE 4

The Duration of Unfilled Pauses Per Syllable by Grade Level

dramatic course of development. Developmental changes are precipitous between kindergarten and second grade, but from then on they are quite leisurely. This is similar to the course of development for the frequency of part-word repetitions. Also, there were significant differences between the sexes in the duration of unfilled pauses at all age levels except 8th grade, the boys using more time than the girls. The figure also shows that the standard deviations parallel the central tendencies closely, as might be expected, the shorter pauses having less room for variation.

Several of the facts just reviewed suggest that the duration of unfilled pauses is an excellent measure of fluency development: (a) it directly influences the rate of speech, (b) it shows strong developmental trends that parallel part-word repetitions, which are a fluency measure of known clinical importance, (c) it distinguishes between the sexes, which we know to be clinically important, and (d) the influence of language complexity on it can be partialled out, as we have done, by dividing each duration by the number of syllables in the subsequent clause, that is, up to the next unfilled pause. The difficulty with unfilled pause duration as a measure of speech fluency is that, even with language complexity partialled out, it is still not independent of language fluency. Children with abnormally long unfilled pauses may be using the extra time to plan language, not speech. In fact, it may be that the duration of unfilled pauses reflects both speech and language fluency together, and this may be why it shows a more rapid developmental pattern and distinguishes between the sexes. Perhaps, when neither speech fluency nor language fluency alone shows a developmental trend or distinguishes between the sexes, the two together may still do so. Perhaps fluency development becomes pathological when speech and language fluency are both delayed.

Despite these uncertainties about how to distinguish between speech and language fluency, it seems clinically feasible to measure the duration of unfilled pauses. Once again, it will be necessary to smooth and interpolate the data to allow for sampling error, and once again, it will be necessary to consider these data in Table II only as a guideline, not a standard. However, it is helpful that, in the case of this measure, Kowal, O'Connell, and Sabin have provided the standard deviations as well as the central tendencies.

The information in Table II can be used to guide clinical decisions about the normality or abnormality of a particular child's pause duration. The standard deviations describe how far

TABLE II

Duration of Unfilled Pauses Per Syllable, By Grade
(Smoothed and Interpolated)

Grade	Mean	Standard Deviation
K	250	197
1	204	152
2	159	107
3	134	82
4	109	58
5	105	57
6	102	56
7	94	51
8	86	46
9	82	40
10	79	33
11	82	34
12	85	34

above or below the group mean a particular child's pause durations are. By subtracting the client's score from the table value and then dividing by the table's standard deviation, a standard score can be derived. But let us not lose sight of the fact that the original data on which our measures are based is too limited to permit more than very cautious conclusions. Also, the kindergarteners and first graders show too much variability to permit any judgment about the degree of deviation from normal. The data suggest that it is normal for children in the early grades to vary widely in this measure.

Speech rate is a complicated, multivariate construct. Speech can be considered at many levels — utterances, words, syllables, sounds, gestures — and the rate of speech means something different at each level.

The highest level is the utterance level, and the length of utterance is related to rate. Of course, longer utterances take longer to produce, but presumably they also contain more information. The question for fluency is whether the amount of time the longer utterance occupies is fully justified by the amount of additional information it contains. The answer clearly is that it is not. There is less information per syllable in longer than in shorter utterances (Starkweather, 1980). As a result, the rate of syllable production is faster in longer than in shorter utterances. This effect makes utterance length an aspect of fluency. Kowal, O'Connell and Sabin (1975) measured the length of utterance by counting the number of syllables per unfilled pause. They found a sharp increase in the length of utterance from kindergarten to second grade, then no change through the next four years, then another sharp increase between sixth and eighth grades and modest increases after that which taper off by senior year. There were no sex differences. The standard deviations show very modest increases throughout the school years, reflecting the fact that, as children's language use matures, they produce a few sentences that are very long. Although utterance length reflects speech fluency, it is confounded with language fluency.

Utterance length is a speech fluency measure of interest even though it is confounded by language fluency, because it is correlated with rate. The rate of speech, in syllables per second, is faster during longer than during shorter utterances. This is apparently because the individual words in longer utterances contain less information as a result of the additional surrounding context that the longer utterance provides (Starkweather, 1980).

The correlation of utterance length with rate increases with age. Disimoni (1974) did an experiment, to which we will be returning later, in which he showed that as children mature the duration of bilabial consonant closure is more likely to be affected by utterance length. Regrettably, he did not report the actual correlations so we can't make any definitive statements about the growth in this relationship. And of course, the study was done with only one speech sound. This relation seems important as far as speech production is concerned because it should be independent of language. Rate, of course, depends on the person's language as well as his speech capacities, and one would expect the additional complexity of longer utterances to require more planning and thus take longer to produce, but this does not happen. The pauses preceding longer utterances may be longer and reflective of language ability, but the speed with which utterances are executed seems to reflect speech production capacity.

It would be helpful in understanding the development of normal fluency to have research focusing on a careful delineation of the relation of speech rate to utterance length, in children of different ages. The magnitude of this relation between stutterers and nonstutterers of different ages should also be investigated. If stutterers showed a higher correlation between length and rate, it might suggest that they are more sensitive to the need for a rapid flow of information than nonstutterers. If stutterers showed a lower correlation between length and rate, it might reflect an inability to produce the faster rates that longer utterances require. Differences in developmental trends between stutterers and nonstutterers would also be instructive. With increasing maturity, normal children become capable of faster movement and show an increasingly larger correlation between length and rate, as Disimoni's data show. For stuttering children, however, the pattern of development may be different. Their increasingly mature skills would tend to strengthen the relation, but the time occupied by stuttering behaviors would increase time pressure, possibly beyond their capacities for rapid movement. More stuttering, and a weaker relation with increasing age, could result. With this data in hand, a stuttering child's capacity for producing speech rapidly could be assessed more thoroughly. Also, it could be that it is through this relation that the length of utterance comes to promote stuttering, i.e., the longer utterances demand more rapid production, and, for whatever reason, the child is not able to produce speech that quickly and stutters as a consequence. It may be that it is not the demand for speed so much as the demand for a change in the rhythm of speech which the increased speed entails that promotes the breakdown in fluency.

Rate can also be assessed at the word level. The word is more of an informational unit than a speech production unit. Consequently, words per minute is a measure of the amount of information a speaker is producing, and this may be independent of the rate at which speech sounds or syllables are produced, as any stutterer knows. When forced to slow down the production of *speech* by metronomic pacing, or even simple instructions, stutterers typically produce more words per minute because so many noninformational, stuttered syllables are left out. This does not mean that words per minute should be ignored. One of the purposes of talking is to transmit information, and measures of stuttering severity are more complete if they include information about the client's ability to transmit information.

The next level at which rate can be assessed is the syllable level. This is clearly the highest (i.e., most molar) level at which speech fluency can be measured without serious confounding by language fluency. For this reason, the number of syllables per second is the basic measure of rate. The rate of speech in adults is 5-6 syllables per second (Walker and Black, 1950). Kowal, O'Connell, and Sabin (1975) measured the rate of speech in syllables per second in their sample of school children telling stories about Snoopy cartoons. Figure 5 shows the development of rate in their sample. It is clear that there is a fairly steady rise in the rate of speech during the school years. Even in the later high school years, the children in this study did not achieve the speech rates reported by other researchers for adults (Walker and Black, 1950; Malecot, Johnston, and Kizziar, 1972). Of course, it is possible that the full adult rate is not reached until after high school. But the data may also be affected by the social context of the testing situation. These children were being assessed in school by authority figures, and may have used a more formal style of speech production, with a slower rate. But these differences do not mean that we cannot use Kowal, O'Connell, and

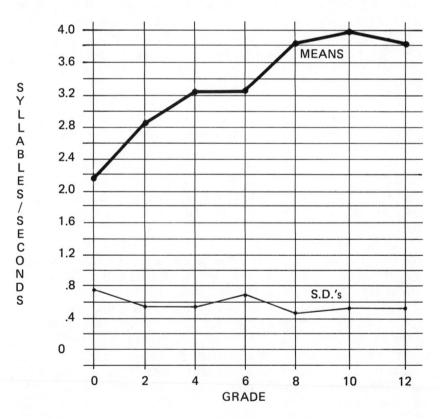

FIGURE 5
The Rate of Speech by Grade Level

Sabin's data for clinical purposes. Indeed, the more formal testing situation they used is far more like the testing situation in a clinic than was the case in the other studies.

One wonders, of course, about the developmental lags that are visible at sixth grade and senior year. Most probably they reflect sampling error. I wonder, though, if they might not also reflect a general uncertainty about the future, the sixth graders because of imminent puberty and the high school seniors because of imminent reality. Things are changing fast at these times of life.

As the mean rate of speech is increasing through the school years, the variability of speech rate remains about the same, and it is rather low. Tiffany (1980) has made an excellent case for the idea that adults talk nearly as fast as they can. This consistently low variability in the rate of speech in school children, which remains low despite a rising central tendency, suggests that children too are probably talking about as fast as their speech mechanisms will allow. Since all of the children in this sample were physiologically normal, it might be presumed that the group was also physiologically similar. Of course, one could also argue that the speech of children occurs at a rate that is consistent across children for social reasons. That is, as with other aspects of language and speech, it is desirable, often necessary, to sound like one's peers. So perhaps there are two forces working for uniformity of speech rate.

In any event, even though these data are not based on large enough, or genuinely standardized samples, we might be able to use them to evaluate the rate of school children's speech. For this purpose, the smoothed and interpolated data are shown in Table III.

Using the smoothed data as a source of guidance in making clinical decisions about the normality of a child's rate of speech would follow the same general principles used before. More than one standard deviation below the mean, for example less than 3 syllables per second for a seventh grader, is quite slow. If we could assume a normal distribution, a score more than one standard deviation below the mean would indicate a child in the lower one-sixth of the distribution. As before, standard scores could be derived by dividing a client's score from the mean for his or her grade and dividing the resulting difference by the standard deviation. It would also be appropriate to use these data as a partial basis for judging the severity of stuttering. We have been too quick in the past, I believe, to judge the severity of stuttering on the simple frequency with which stuttering

TABLE III

Speech Rate in Schoolchildren in Syllables Per Second
(Smoothed and Interpolated)

Grade	Mean	Standard Deviation
K	2.33	.70
1	2.56	.64
2	2.78	.58
3	2.97	.57
4	3.15	.56
5	3.28	.58
6	3.40	.59
7	3.57	.57
8	3.74	.55
9	3.83	.53
10	3.92	.52
11	3.90	.52
12	3.88	.52

behaviors occur. The rate at which stutterers are able to produce syllables is another important piece of diagnostic information. It provides some information about a client's ability to communicate. Other factors, of course, need also to be considered. But in the past this important measure has often been neglected in the evaluation of stuttering.

It should be clear that, as with continuity, a large sample study of speech rate in children should be a major priority of research in normal fluency. Until those results are in, we can cautiously use these data.

The next level at which rate can be assessed is the phone level, i.e., the number of phones per second can be measured. This measure reflects almost exactly the same processes seen in the syllables per second measure. As long as a large enough sample is obtained so that there is enough variety, the phone rate will be reflected in the syllabic rate, which is easier to derive. It might be worth noting at this point, however, that different types of syllables are produced faster or slower, depending on the types of sounds they are composed of, which is why a large sample of speech is necessary in assessing rate. Specifically, syllables that begin with consonants are produced more quickly than syllables that begin with vowels (MacKay, 1974). The type of sound initiating the syllable is a more important factor than the number of phones in it.

The next level at which rate can be assessed is the segmental level, the level of the phone itself — not how many phones can be produced per second, but how much time elapses during the production of a single phone. This measure is not derivable from the number of syllables produced per second because of the phenomenon of coarticulation. Speakers may do two different things to increase the number of syllables (or phones) they produce per second — they may move more rapidly, or they may increase the amount of coarticulatory overlap between adjacent gestures. There are constraints within which this decision must operate: (1) the speed of movement is limited to the speaker's physiological capacity, (2) certain sounds and certain features of sounds depend specifically on the speed of movement or on the duration of time between events — consonant-vowel transitions depend on the rate with which movement occurs, and voiced-voiceless distinctions depend on the relative timing of consonantal release and voice onset, and (3) adjacent gestures can be overlapped only so much before the loss to intelligibility is too great. However, within these constraints, speech can be speeded up or slowed down by either of these two strategies.

I wish I could say that there have been extensive studies of the duration of speech sounds and of coarticulation in normal children, but such data are rare. In a few studies, however, it has been shown that anticipatory coarticulation is more common in older than in younger speakers (Thompson and Hixon, 1979) and that the extent of anticipatory coarticulation is greater in adults than in four-year-olds (Kent and Forner, 1980). Kent (1983) summarizes these and other data as showing that speech development "serves to produce motor patterns that are rapid, efficient, and highly anticipatory." (p. 75) A few studies have also been done on the duration of phones in children of different ages. One of these was done by Disimoni (1974). This researcher asked ten children at each of three age groups — 3, 6, and 9 years — to produce the sound /p/ surrounded by the vowel /i/. They produced this VCV utterance alone, and they also produced it as part of a sentence frame. The purpose of the experiment was to see if the effect of utterance length on sound duration, known to occur in adults, was also present in the speech of children at different ages. It was, but the more interesting part of the data is the changes in central tendency and variability that occurred with development. In both the short and the long utterances, the mean duration of /p/ declined with age, and the standard deviation for this measure also declined. There is clearly a developmental trend in the duration of speech sounds accompanied by a diminishing variability. This suggests that the child is gaining control over speech production at the same time as fluency is increasing.

Another study was done by Tassiello (1975). She asked 30 seven year olds and 30 five year olds to respond to picture stimuli and produce words beginning with /s/ but from a variety of vowel environments. Since there were no differences in the duration of /s/ in different environments in this study, the data was pooled. The seven year olds showed significantly briefer durations of /s/ than the five-year-olds. Standard deviations for the five year olds were 14.11, those for the seven-year-olds were 11.07. Neither of these two sets of data are sufficient to use in clinical evaluations, but at least they demonstrate a developmental trend in the ability of children to produce speech sounds of briefer duration and to do this with increasing control.

There is an important research need in this area too. Umeda (1975; 1977) has done some exquisitely detailed studies of the duration of speech sounds in samples of adult spontaneous speech, and documented many of the contextual variables which determine the duration of individual sounds. This is important because, as it turns out, the contextual effects that influence the duration of speech sounds are the same as the linguistic locations that predict stuttering — word and clause boundaries, syllabic stress, word length, word frequency, and word type. It is useful to think of these variations in the duration of speech sounds as minute variations in the rate of speech. Rate speeds up after a pause, then gradually slows down to the next pause. Superimposed on that slow change in rate are briefer fluctuations in rate that occur as the speaker moves from one word to the next. And in addition, the extra duration that is given to the sounds in a stressed syllable may be seen as a very brief slowing of the speech rate. These small fluctuations in rate make demands on the rhythmic control of speech, and will lead us into the following discussion of rhythm. First, we need to recognize that there is need for a study on the speech of children, comparable in method to Umeda's work on adult spontaneous speech. This is a formidable undertaking, but it would pay off by increasing our understanding of the effects of language variables on fluency in children. It may be that children find it less easy to make adjustments in rhythm and timing, which are associated with syntactic structure. Stuttering children, or children who are likely to become stutterers, may find it even harder than normal children.

IV. The Development of Rhythm and Prosody

The first words of babies are arhythmic. It takes more than one word to establish the variable that we call speech rhythm. Speech rhythm can be defined in a number of different ways, but any definition will have to be based on the pattern with which stressed and unstressed syllables occur. There are actually several levels of stress, but we can make our discussion much easier without sacrificing any vital information by considering only two levels — stressed and unstressed. The preceding sentence would be scanned into two stress levels as follows:

--/--/-/--/---/--/--/---/--/--/---//---/-/---/---/--/-/-//-(pause)/-/-.

It is immediately apparent that there is regularity, or structure, in this pattern. Stressed syllables seem to alternate with two or three unstressed syllables. Occasionally there is a single unstressed syllable, and more rarely none between stressed syllables. There is a tendency, not visible in this kind of scan, for unstressed syllables to be shortened even further when there are several of them in a row, and there is also a tendency to slow down when two stressed syllables occur together. These effects make the structure of speech rhythm more evident in acoustic than in graphic form. In English, we try to achieve a steady rhythm between stressed syllables, and we perceive such a rhythm, even though in actual speech, the rhythm is less than regular (Fowler, 1979; Tuller and Fowler, 1980).

When children first begin to say words, they often produce bisyllabic words that do not contain unstressed syllables. Since unstressed syllables are briefer it may be that the child, who is just beginning to develop his ability to produce speech, isn't able to move fast enough or isn't able to adjust the relative timing of movements, to make unstressed syllables. Or perhaps the child can't hear the distinction well enough at first to model his own speech after it. Whatever the reason, children at the two and three morpheme level of development often substitute stressed for unstressed syllables. The most common pattern is for a nearby, usually adjacent, stressed syllable to be used instead of the unstressed one, as in "rayray" for "raisins." Sometimes some of the sounds from the unstressed syllable are incorporated into the substitution. Often, a string of two or three unstressed syllables is replaced by one stressed one, as in "pumjums" for "pajamas," or "tayto" for "tomato." Then gradually, the ability to produce unstressed syllables develops. By the time they reach the four morpheme level, most children are using the right number of syllables and have a clear appreciation of speech rhythm, even though their phonological processes are still developing. At this point they produce words like "ferigerator" for "refrigerator," "themoneber" for "thermometer," and sing "My Country Tennessee." They may not have the lyric, but they've got rhythm.

There is not much information about the development of stress contrast in children's speech, and what work has been done is not seen from the point of view of fluency. It would be useful to document this developmental sequence more fully. Since stuttering occurs almost exclusively on stressed syllables, it seems important to understand how the distinction between stressed and unstressed syllables develops. Also, it is typically at just this same point in development that some children begin to produce long part-word repetitions. Children are able to discriminate stressed from unstressed syllables from birth (Spring and Dale, 1977). It would be interesting to know the details of the development of stress contrast production, from the production of the first unstressed syllable, to the ability to produce two unstressed syllables in a row, then three, and so on. We know so little about this area that it is hard even to be sure how to go about making the observations. It would be interesting to discover what kinds of underlying physiological capacities the perception and production of stress contrast depends upon. Is it just a matter of coordination and speed, or is there an underlying oscillator that has to be operative?

The rhythm of speech seems to be directly related to fluency in three different ways: (1) unstressing increases rate, (2) the structure of rhythm makes it easier to produce speech faster, and (3) rhythm is related to gesture, which is related to fluency. Let's look at these three relations one at a time.

First, on a rather superficial level, the unstressed syllable is briefer than the stressed one and so saves the speaker a little time. This may seem insignificant, but it adds up quickly. With all the other things we do to produce information at a rapid rate, unstressing may serve the same function. Not that speakers consciously unstress syllables so as to gain time, but rather that the language has evolved in a way that maximizes its basic utility — the transmission of information.

The second way that rhythm is related to rate has to do with the structure of rhythm. Martin (1972), in a classic paper, shows how the rhythm of speech provides a temporal structure, which is conventionally held among speakers of a language. Earlier, we described the structure of rhythm in English as the tendency for stressed syllables to occur within a certain time frame. This is a convention that speakers and listeners share, and it enables listeners to anticipate, in a probabilistic way, when a stressed syllable is likely to occur. Although that may not seem like very much information to go on, it nevertheless makes a slight reduction in the uncertainty with which listeners must anticipate future speech events. As a result, listeners can decode a stream of language somewhat faster for having a small part of the information beforehand. Since listeners can decode a little faster, speakers can talk a little faster. In this way rhythm serves rate and fluency by reducing slightly the uncertainty of timing in heard speech.

There is, however, another way in which rhythm serves fluency and rate. Since the structure of a language's rhythm is a convention, a given that reduces uncertainty about *when* stressed syllables are going to occur, it not only helps the listener comprehend, it also helps the speaker produce strings of syllables by narrowing the range of possibilities and consequently reducing the uncertainty. It reduces the uncertainty of *when* a movement is to be initiated. This is evident in the fluency stutterers show when they speak in time to a rhythmic signal and time each syllable with the beat. The signal then totally determines when the syllable is to be produced, so that there is no uncertainty at all. So the rhythmic structure of language helps the speaker by providing a little information about when to initiate a movement.

Finally rhythm is related to gesture and gesture is related to fluency. It has been shown in a number of studies that human beings tend to gesture and move in synchrony with the syllabic rhythm of their own utterance (Duchan, Oliva, and Lindner, 1979; Condon and Ogston, 1966). Certain types of gestures are made simultaneously with stressed syllables, sometimes for extreme emphasis, but nonemphatic gestures are also often in synchrony with speech syllables. It isn't difficult to think of many examples where a complex sequence of movements is initiated simultaneously with another movement that is anatomically different. The concert pianist bows her head as she begins a difficult phrase. The "entrainment" of a second movement seems to assist the timing and execution of the first. So, it may be that the gesture facilitates fluency. Of course, we have known for a long time that stutterers could speak more fluently if they timed their speech so that the stressed syllables coincided with hand gestures or other body movements, and many stutterers discover this phenomenon for themselves and use it to get through tight spots. But it may be that gesture facilitates fluency in nonstutterers too. A dissertation at Columbia by Hoffman (1968) suggests the possibility. Hoffman restricted his subjects so that they could not move their hands while they talked. He recorded their speech and analyzed it later and compared it with the same subjects talking on similar topics without having their hands restrained. It took the subjects longer to say what they wanted to when they couldn't move their hands, although they didn't produce more disfluencies. Nevertheless, it seems likely that gesturing facilitates fluency.

This raises some interesting questions with regard to children. Gesture, of course, is theorized to play a role in the emergence of language in children. What kind of role does it play in the emergence of fluency, if any? There is no data about speech rhythm that we can use to answer this question. Nor is there any data that will guide us in making clinical decisions about normal and abnormal fluency in children. Certainly, we should look for rhythmic structure that is unusual. But we should also listen to children's speech for patterns of stressed and unstressed syllables that sound unusual. We should think about a child's use of gesture and question whether it is serving speech production appropriately. There is little that we can do but ask questions until research provides some more answers. Here are some specific research questions about speech rhythm in children which, in addition to those already mentioned, would provide useful information: 1. Do children with disfluent speech or slow rate show different rhythmic capacities? 2. Exactly when and how does the ability to produce one, two, or three consecutive unstressed syllables develop? 3. What is the relationship of gesture to speech rhythm in children? 4. Can children whose hands are restrained talk as fluently or quickly as when they are not restrained? 5. Are there correlations between speech rhythm variables and rate in developing children? 6. Do children, when they are asked to talk faster, show greater coarticulatory overlap the way adults do (Gay, 1978) or do they just try to move faster? Or can't they do either as well?

V. Developmental Changes in Speech Effort

The last dimension of fluency is effort. Intuitively, we recognize that speech that requires excessive effort is not fluent. Fluent speech is relaxed and easy. There are two types of effort—muscular effort and mental effort. Both of these types are important as far as fluency is concerned. For obvious reasons, more is known about the former than the latter. The muscular effort of disfluent speech is apparent in the struggling, forcing, and tension that clinicians, or any listeners can see and hear. The mental effort is less evident, but is commonly reported and is a serious part of the problem. Stutterers spend much of their thought on matters related to their stuttering. They may search for words that do not start with a worrisome sound. They may search for a way to express their intentions without using a word or phrase that contains semantic features associated with former stuttering episodes. Many stutterers report intense scanning of their listeners for reactions to their stuttering behavior. Much of the time they are simply assessing the possibilities for stuttering in the words that are up ahead lying in wait. Self-assessments also occupy stutterers' thoughts. Reactions like the following are common — "That was a bad one." "I wonder how I'll do on that word." "Finally, I got through that mess." But even during periods of relative fluency, thoughts related to stuttering still occur. "I'm pretty fluent today." "I wonder why I didn't stutter on that word; I always do." "I've been speaking for hours and I haven't stuttered once; how long can this last?" A client of mine recently commented on all this activity by saying, "You really have to be smart to stutter. There is so much to do it's like playing three games of chess simultaneously." In normal speakers, very little thought is devoted to speech production. It runs mostly on automatic pilot, and this is an important quality of speech, for speech production is supposed to serve the communicative goal of getting the speaker's thoughts into the listener's head, and the speaker cannot be preoccupied with the details of speech production and think clearly, swiftly, and creatively.

An interesting experiment by Ladefoged, Silverstein, and Papcun (1973) shows that the thinking time that is devoted to speech production occurs prior to utterance. These researchers asked speakers to interrupt speech production and do something else at a certain signal. The speakers found it difficult to stop what they were doing only in the few moments before utterance, indicating that the time just before utterance involved some concentration. Since the speech task the subjects were being asked to perform was a memorized sentence, it could be presumed that their thinking time was devoted to speech production. Another study by Linebaugh (1975) demonstrated that there is a suppression of alpha wave activity in the speech hemisphere just prior to utterance in normal speakers. Alpha activity is associated with a resting state of the brain, so the speech centers become active, as one might expect, just before speech begins. One can conclude that some thought is required just before an utterance to plan its execution, but once this planning is accomplished the utterance is executed automatically. When this idea is put together with the data reported earlier on the length of unfilled pauses in children, which tend to shorten as the child matures, it appears that children spend more time thinking just before they produce an utterance, and that the amount of thought required to plan an utterance decreases as the child develops.

There are some data that bear on muscular and mental effort in adults. These data suggest that the sense of muscular effort is related to intra-oral air pressure. In producing sounds we oppose forces by causing air to flow and then constricting the airway. It is natural that this opposition of forces should feel effortful. However, it should then be recognized that the sensation of effort is probably not associated only with intra-oral air pressure but also, perhaps even more, with subglottal air pressure. Stutterers often report the exertion of effort as associated with the building up of pressure, either within the mouth or below the glottis. Also, they often report, during therapy, a sense of easing of effort and a sensation of speaking more freely as they learn to keep these pressures down to lower levels.

Effort can also be measured more directly through electromyography. Several studies (Freeman and Ushijima, 1978; Shapiro, 1980) have shown that muscle activity is higher during stuttering than during fluent speech, so it seems appropriate to think of muscular effort as an aspect, indeed an important aspect, of fluency. There have been no studies that I know of in which the muscle activity levels of normal children during speech were reported. The technique is not one that lends itself particularly well to clinical application anyway.

It is worth noting that the two types of effort are associated with different aspects of speech production. Thinking time occurs just before utterance and is by inference associated with planning speech (and language). Muscular effort, what there is of it, occurs during utterance. So mental effort is for planning, muscular effort for execution. The distinction between planning and execution is an important one. Borden (1982) recently reported an experiment in which stutterers and nonstutterers were compared in their planning and execution time for speech and non-speech tasks. The results are rather complicated, but it would be fair to describe them as indicating that stutterers, even when given extra planning time, still execute a series of movements more slowly than nonstutterers. At least, this is true for severe stutterers. It seems that planning and execution are different activities, and it may not be possible to trade off one with the other, at least for stutterers. This is related to an idea expressed earlier — that pauses in speech may actually increase rate by allowing the speaker to plan a little more completely the coordination of movements that are then executed. Then they can be executed more quickly. Whether this is true or not remains to be seen. Borden's data suggest that if such a trade-off exists, it is less available for use by severe stutterers than for nonstutterers.

Although there are no data related to the amount of effort used by children in producing speech, it seems likely that children may use more effort than adults. Their speech sounds as if it is produced with more effort. If that intuition is correct, then in this dimension too, children are less fluent speakers than adults. This intuition, however, may be derived simply from the fact that they talk more slowly. But that inference is appropriate because rate and effort are related.

When speakers are asked to talk more quickly, intra-oral air pressure is reduced (Arkebauer, 1964), contrary to what might be expected, so rapid speech feels less effortful. The important point, however, is that effort is greater in slower speech. Probably, the additional muscular effort involved in building up higher levels of intra-oral air pressure takes additional time. Also, it takes additional time for this additional air pressure to be dissipated. Although there are no data, it seems reasonable to suppose that the same relationship holds true for subglottal air pressure. I would guess that it is also true for more direct measures of effort, such as electromyographic activity.

It is interesting to speculate about the possible relationship of gesture to speech effort. There isn't any real evidence, but it is possible that the synchronous gestures increases fluency by reducing the effort involved in executing a sequence of movements. Specifically, gestures may make the initiation of the sequence less effortful. When dealing with a coordinated set of movements like speech, the approach that seems to have evolved is to spend some time planning the sequence and then executing it. Again, the analogy I like is that of the football team huddling to plan a play and then executing it. An important part of such a strategy is determining precisely the moment at which the execution sequence is supposed to begin. The synchronous gesture in speech, then, is like the hike signal — an external event that gets all the parts to start moving at the same time. Of course in speech, the parts may not actually begin moving at the same time, but the movement of each part has to be coordinated relative to points in time, and the synchronous gesture can assist in achieving this. Kelso, Tuller, and Harris (1983) have shown that functionally related movements tend to become "entrained" or synchronized. They asked subjects to say a word repeatedly, alternating stressed and unstressed productions and to tap their fingers at the same time but to keep the magnitude of each finger tap equal, i.e., not to let the simultaneously alternating stress of the speech task influence the steady tap, tap of the finger. Despite instructions not to, the subjects showed finger taps of greater magnitude during production of stressed words. It is hard not to entrain one movement with another related one. It may consequently be *easier* to make a movement if another one is entrained with it. Thus, synchronous hand, head, foot, or body movements may make speech production easier.

These ideas are not sufficiently detailed or specifically related to disfluency to be applied to clinical evaluations about individual children. However, we can and should be aware of the ease with which children produce speech and evaluate their speech as less fluent when it seems as though they are using more muscular effort or thinking time than seems normal. We can compensate for the lack of empirical verification of effort by using the known relationship of effort to rate. If rate is slow, it can be presumed that effort is high. Furthermore, an analysis of the factors that contribute to slow rate may make it possible to distinguish between rate that is slowed by excessive planning time and rate that is slowed by excessive muscular effort during execution. Planning time will be reflected in unfilled pauses that are longer than normal. Execution time will be reflected in a low output of syllables per second between pauses. Consequently, a profile of a child, based on the data presented earlier, would differentiate between these two aspects of speech rate. A child who shows unfilled pauses that are longer than normal but executes syllables in a normal amount of time could be described as disfluent in the planning of speech, whereas a child whose unfilled pause durations were normal but whose output of syllables per second was slow could be described as disfluent in the execution of speech movements. It would also be helpful to note, and if possible record on videotape for careful analysis, the synchrony of gestures with speech movements.

Summary and Conclusions

This chapter has dealt with the measures that need to be taken in evaluating the fluency of young speakers. Briefly, these measures are the amount of time taken up by interruptions in the continuity of speech, the proportion of discontinuities that are of an immature type, the duration of pauses, the number of syllables produced per second, and the number of syllables produced per pause. The chapter has also suggested the need for research efforts in the areas of rate, rhythm, and effort of speech production. Lacking a firm empirical basis for making a precise determination of when speech is abnormally disfluent, we can say that fluency is deviant when speech is produced with effort, when speech is more discontinuous than normal, or when the discontinuities are immature, when the rhythm of speech is atypical, or when it is not serving the speaker by making speech production easier. The operationalization of these variables will have to wait for further research on the development of fluency in children.

References

Arkebauer, H. J., *A Study of Intra-Oral Air Pressure Associated with the Production of Selected Consonants.* Doctoral dissertation, State University of Iowa, 1964.

Borden, G., *Initiation Versus Execution Time During Manual and Oral Counting by Stutterers.* Convention address, ASHA, 1982.

Carrow, E., *Test for Auditory Comprehension of Language.* Austin, Texas: Urban Research Grove, 1973.

Condon, W. S., and Ogston, W. D., "Soundfilm Analysis of Normal and Pathological Behavioral Patterns," *Journal of Nervous and Mental Diseases,* 143, 338-347, 1966.

Davis, D., "The Relation of Repetitions in the Speech of Young Children to Certain Measures of Language Maturity and Situational Factors: Part I, *Journal of Speech Disorders,* 4, 303-318, 1939.

Disimoni, F. G., "Preliminary Study of Certain Timing Relationships in the Speech of Stutterers," *Journal of the Acoustical Society of America,* 56, 695-696, 1974.

Duchan, J., Oliva, J., and Lindner, R., "Performative Acts Defined by Synchrony Among Intonational Verbal and Nonverbal Systems in a One-and-a-half-year-old Child," *Sign Language Studies,* 22, 75-88, 1979.

Fillmore, C. J., "On Fluency," *Individual Differences in Language Ability and Language Behavior,* Pp. 85-101. New York: Academic Press, 1979.

Fowler, C., " 'Perceptual Centers' in Speech Production and Perception," *Perception and Psychophysics,* 2, 375-388, 1979.

Haynes, W. O., and Hood, S. B., "Language and Disfluency Variables in Normal Speaking Children From Discrete Chronological Age Groups," *Journal of Fluency Disorders,* 2, 57-74, 1977.

Hoffman, S. P., *An Empirical Study of Representational Hand Movements.* Doctoral dissertation, New York University, 1968.

Johnson, W., *The Onset of Stuttering.* Minneapolis: University Minneapolis Press, 1961.

Johnson, W., *Speech Handicapped School Children.* New York: Harper, 1956.

Kelso, J. A. S., Tuller, B., and Harris, K. S., "A 'Dynamic Pattern' Perspective on the Control and Coordination of Movement," in MacNeilage, P. F., *Speech Production.* New York: Springer-Verlag, 1983.

Kent, R. D., "The Segmental Organization of Speech," in MacNeilage, P. F., *The Production of Speech.* New York: Springer-Verlag, 1983.

Kent, R. D., and Forner, L. L., "Speech Segment Durations in Sentence Recitations by Children and Adults," *Journal of Phonetics,* 8, 157-168, 1980.

Kline, M. L., and Starkweather, C. W., *Receptive and Expressive Language Performance in Young Stutterers.* Convention address, American Speech and Hearing Association, 1979. Abstract in *ASHA,* 21, 797, 1979.

Kowal, S., O'Connell, D. C., and Sabin, E. F., "Development of Temporal Patterning and Vocal Hesitations in Spontaneous Narratives," *Journal of Psycholinguistic Research,* 4, 195-207, 1975.

Ladefoged, P., Silverstein, R., and Papcun, G., "Interruptibility of Speech," *Journal of the Acoustical Society of America,* 54, 1105-1108, 1973.

Linebaugh, C., *Interhemispheric Asymmetries in the Contingent Negative Variation and Cerebral Dominance for Speech Production*. Doctoral dissertation, Temple University, 1975.

MacKay, D. G., "Aspects of the Syntax of Behavior: Syllable structure and Speech Rate," *Quarterly Journal of Experimental Psychology*, 26, 642-657, 1974.

Malecot, A., Johnston, R., and Kizziar, P. A., "Syllabic Rate and Utterance Length in French," *Phonetica*, 26, 235-251, 1972.

Martin, J., "Rhythmic (Hierarchical) Versus Serial Structure in Speech and Other Behavior," *Psychological Review*, 79, 487-509, 1972.

Sheehan, J. G., and Martyn, M. M., "Spontaneous Recovery from Stuttering," *Journal of Speech and Hearing Research*, 9, 279-289, 1970.

Spring, D. R., and Dale, P. S., "Discrimination of Linguistic Stress in Early Infancy," *Journal of Speech and Hearing Research*, 20, 224-232, 1977.

Starkweather, C. W., "Speech Fluency and Its Development in Normal Children," in Lass, N. (Ed.), *Speech and Language: Advances in Basic Research and Practice*, Volume 4, 1981.

Tassiello, M., *Duration of /s/ in Five and Seven Year Olds*. Master of Arts thesis, Hunter College, 1975.

Thompson, A. E., and Hixon, T. J., "Nasal Air Flow During Normal Speech Production," *Cleft Palate Journal*, 16, 412-430, 1979.

Tiffany, W. R., "The Effects of Syllable Structure on Diadochokinetic and Reading Rates," *Journal of Speech and Hearing Research*, 23, 894-908, 1980.

Tuller, B., and Fowler, C., "Some Articulatory Correlates of Perceptual Isochrony," *Perception and Psychophysics*, 27, 277-283, 1980.

Umeda, N., "Vowel Duration in American English," *Journal of the Acoustical Society of America*, 58, 434-445, 1975.

Umeda, N., "Consonant Duration in American English," *Journal of the Acoustical Society of America*, 61, 846-858, 1977.

Walker, C., and Black, J., *The Intrinsic Intensity of Oral Phrases*, Joint Project Report No. 2. Pensacola, Florida: Naval Air Station, U. S. Naval School of Aviation Medicine, 1950.

Wexler, K., "Developmental Disfluency in 2, 4, and 6-year-old Boys in Neutral and Stress Situations," *Journal of Speech and Hearing Research*, 25, 229-234, 1982.

Yairi, E., "Disfluencies of Normally Speaking Two-year-old Children," *Journal of Speech and Hearing Research*, 24, 490-495, 1981.

chapter five

Toward a Therapy Assessment Procedure for Treating Stuttering in Children

Roger J. Ingham, Ph.D.
University of California
Santa Barbara

Introduction

There are many ways of addressing this topic, but I think they boil down to two broad approaches. The first is to review the stuttering literature to find what has been done in the way of assessment and then pass judgement on its worth. The other way, which I think bypasses at least a modicum of controversy, is to try to identify what clinicians and clinical researchers might accept as necessary components in a stuttering assessment system—that is, one that would permit internally and externally valid conclusions to be reached about the operation of a therapy process. I am certainly not sure that this common ground can be found, and maybe it is presumptuous to even assume the existence of such an Elysian Field. Nevertheless, it does seem to be the less problem-filled approach to this difficult task.

A few years ago (Ingham and Lewis, 1978) I thought that the only way clinical researchers would ever be satisfied with the reliability and validity of data from any stuttering treatment would be for it to include 24-hour, covert, audio-visual recordings made over a respectable interval of time embracing the before, during, and after periods of treatment. Now as I look at the issue, I think I was far too conservative. Nowadays, I think that these recordings would have to be accompanied by fiber-optic view of the larynx (if the subject has one), EMG and EEG traces, air-flow analyses, spectrographic records of Voice Initiation Times (VIT's), Voice Termination Times (VTT's), and Voice Onset Times (VOT's), phonation measures, plus, of course, measures of linguistic structure. Then we would be remiss if we didn't include perceptual analyses of speech quality, and a nice variety of questionnaires that tap the subject's judgements, especially their attitudes toward communication. Perhaps for good measure we should also have assessments made by the parents and "significant others" to ensure that their needs are also satisfied. Yet, even then we would not want our clients' uncontrollable expectations of therapy success to clutter up our evaluations; we would want them to have a twin stutterer (preferably monozygotic) who should receive a parallel package of assessments but without the luxury of our preferred treatment. In short, for some of us, defining sufficient reliability and validity in stuttering assessment is probably like defining sufficiency for many of our baser needs; we can't get enough of them and they certainly benefit from variety.

Of course, what this reflects is the unsatisfactory level of construct validity among our present procedures for assessing stuttering. To a large extent, this is linked with the problems that Starkweather (1980) and others have described in defining a measure of normally fluent speech. For as long as we continue to have difficulties in finding the necessary and sufficient components for determining normal fluency, then we are probably going to continue to have difficulties in measuring or even recognizing this ultimate goal of stuttering therapy. So, almost at the outset, our search for a common set of assessment procedures is destined to failure; but perhaps not total failure. For that may largely depend upon what purpose we expect our assessment procedure to fulfill.

We might all agree that any therapy assessment procedure should have some links with a therapy purpose. I believe that it is at this point that we have managed to create a measurement mess that is as confusing to clinicians as it is to clinical researchers—let alone our clients. At one extreme, we have those therapy procedures that seemingly regard speech behavior as an incidental element in treatment, while at the other we have treatments that regard anything *but* speech behavior as irrelevant information. The legacy of this is a remarkable tentativeness in our therapy literature toward specifying criteria of success and failure in stuttering therapy. Perhaps I can manage to step over some parts of this problem by asserting that in the case of children, stuttering therapy should be primarily concerned with altering speech behavior and very much less concerned with nonspeech behavior variables, although it certainly should not ignore them entirely.

Whatever else we disagree about, I am certain that we do agree that stuttering is a variable behavior, and that any assessment procedure must take account of that variability. One fundamental reason for doing so in a therapy context is simply to insure that our evaluation of therapy progress or outcome is not confounded by the untreated variability in the subject's stuttering behavior. Fortunately, we now have recourse to some useful therapy evaluation formats that are based upon an analysis of variability. They also have the advantage of dealing with some common concerns in clinical practice such as accountability, decision making, and outcome evaluation. I refer to formats based on the time series quasi-experimental designs (Hersen and Barlow, 1976) that are typically used in single-subject research. These designs not only have the advantage of helping the clinician to isolate the effects of treatments, but they also provide for a continuing evaluation of the therapy process. They are not only the most powerful designs that we have available to determine sources of within-subject variability, but they are the only ones that will permit us to discern whether a treatment produces generalized changes in the object of treatment.

The strength, or internal and external validity, of these designs in this context depends on repeated data collection within and beyond the therapy setting. It is also enhanced by data that are collected at clinically relevant intervals before, during, and after treatment. In short, what I wish to commend as a foundation stone for erecting a general therapy assessment format is an integration of the familiar multibaseline and ABA designs. But in order to even begin to make this general design clinically viable, and thereby an acceptable vehicle for assessment, we must find some agreement on the frequency, duration, and content of the measures that need to be entered in the format's design.

Necessary Conditions
for Time-Series Assessments
in Stuttering Therapy

At the very outset I would contend that we need a minimum of audio-recorded speech behavior within relevant speaking conditions. Without either we have no reasonably reliable basis for establishing the variability of stuttering within and across conditions that are reputed to influence that variability. It would be useful if these could be supplemented by video recordings, but our technology is not sufficiently developed for viable field video recordings (such recordings would certainly improve our capacity to measure the variability and severity of stuttering moments as well as stuttering frequency).

The choice of the situations in which these measurements should be made will be conditioned by their recordability as much as their validity. To assist the recording process, we now have available exceedingly small, good quality micro-cassette recorders that should not be beyond the resources of a clinic or, indeed, many clients. They can be worn comfortably and equipped with remote hand controls that make it simple to record in most situations. The choice of recordable assessment situations, especially for children, will present some complicated, but not unsolvable, difficulties. There are some logical choices; with parents, peers, and significant others in the child's speaking environment. However, the validity of these situations may be aided by two other factors; the child's choice of "difficult" but recordable situations, and the relative frequency with which these situations occur. These additional considerations should certainly be included within the decision-base that is used to choose samples from the child's environment. One logical starting point for deciding the sample sizes is that they should reflect the typical speaking time that occurs in any of the settings. If the child's speaking time with his parents occupies more than 50% of estimated speaking times (speaking time could be derived with reasonable precision from logs kept by the child or the child's parents), then this should be represented proportionately in the sampling time. Proportional representation certainly carries the right spirit for agreement, if not for validity.

Reaching an agreeable decision about the frequency and duration of samples in a repeated measures assessment design involves at least three considerations; identifying variability, establishing that a treatment is "working," and data management. However, taking account of these considerations in a generally acceptable therapy format is like putting together a jigsaw puzzle that has the pieces shaped and made by special interest groups whose members can never agree. And we certainly have plenty of those groups. Nevertheless I shall try.

Perhaps the first puzzle piece should come from the ranks of clinical researchers who have argued at length over the minimum number of data points that are needed to reflect variability. For compromise purposes I will defer to the much-used text by Hersen and Barlow (1976) that suggests that there should be at least three or four "data points" in any phase of an evaluation design employing data trend comparisons. If we accept the seemingly small number of four, does this translate into four consecutive days, once every four weeks, or perhaps, once every four months? I think that this piece of the puzzle should come from our overworked clinicians in the field. It relates to the frequency with which treatment is offered and the interval of time needed to convince our peers that treatment efficacy has been established. Presumably the object of treatment is to show that reductions or increases (in whatever the behavior) unambiguously differ from those found during a baserate period. We are therefore faced with our second consideration; making a decision about what will be regarded as a significant treatment benefit. But allow me to defer the search for that puzzle piece for a moment. The third, and most overlooked factor, is the sheer task of assessing data obtained from audio-recordings, and the subject's ability to obtain such recordings. Actually, the indeterminate number and size of our puzzle's pieces start to take some shape at this point. For much of their shape depends on a decision about frequency of therapy contact. If conventional individual therapy is used as a first point of reference, then it is usually a maximum of an hour twice weekly. Within that time, or between these times, we need to permit a sufficient interval to process data.

Let us now try to find a suitable time-frame that can be used to decide whether therapy is beneficial or not beneficial. Seemingly, we immediately face a veritable Pandora's Box—comparing different therapies and their effects. Well, our view into the box is not as daunting as we might expect. We can now take advantage of a body of therapy literature that should help us estimate the rate of change in target behaviors from successfully treated clients. Indeed, if that literature cannot be used for this purpose then it has virtually no external validity (Birnbrauer, 1981). At the very least, it should teach us the rate of change in stuttering to expect if a client is responsive to a particular treatment. For example, if our treatment of choice was one of the response contingent procedures, then perhaps we should expect a very much less dramatic decline in stuttering frequency than would be the case with rhythm or any of the ever-growing list of variants of prolonged speech. On the other hand, the relevant target behavior for these speech pattern techniques may well be restoration of normal speech rate which, of course, would extend the time by which treatment responsiveness should be determined.

There is no reason to skirt the "treatment effect time" issue with generalities since our treatment literature, at least that which provides single-subject data from children (12 years and younger), is able to be summarized for this purpose. I have prepared a separate summary of these studies from which it is possible to estimate the point at which stuttering or disfluencies (sometimes "dysfluencies") decreased by 50% from baserate in "successful" clients. I have chosen 50% as a compromise indicator of responsiveness (what could be more of a compromise than 50%?). It shows that young children, five years or younger, treated by a response-contingent punishment schedule reached a 50% reduction in a target behavior by a maximum of about three treatment hours. For older children, the maximum was one and a half treatment hours. The GILCU studies are more difficult to translate unless we accept half the time taken to reach the final target behavior as equivalent to 50% improvement. This turns out to be a maximum of about 30 hours—although roughly 12½ hours might be more reasonable since the 30 hour response rate appears to be an extreme score.

So, how does this information help us with our treatment format puzzle? It helps if we accept that treatment effect time and baserate periods need to be of similar duration if plausible comparisons are to be made between the variability in both phases of our therapy format. Therefore, in the case of the response-contingent stimulation techniques, it would suggest that twice-weekly hourly sessions might be preceded by at least two weeks of twice-weekly baserate data. This would probably be the minimum period. The maximum period, based upon all the summarized treatments would be around six weeks of twice-weekly data collection. Coincidentally, Andrews and Harvey (1981) reported that pretreatment measures of speech behavior in groups of stutterers, that included children, did not show substantial changes over six weeks. Consequently, if we split the difference between the maximum and minimum intervals, we should emerge with a reasonably viable—even agreeable—baserate interval. And if this part of the puzzle fits our purpose, then around four weeks of twice-weekly recordings should precede hourly therapy sessions held twice-weekly.

Thus the logical consequence of our assessment design would suggest that the treatment phase for almost all of the current data-based treatments should not exceed about 12 hours before a decision is made as to whether the treatment should continue or be changed. Presumably, quite discernable trends in relevant data (or, data measures resembling those used in the reported studies) may be expected between the second and fourth hour of treatment.

Another issue concerns the point at which treatment should cease. In the context of the broad format developed thus far, perhaps stability over four treatment weeks might be a reasonable criteria. This would insure that the subject's improved performance has been sustained long enough to determine that it unambiguously differs from pre-treatment performance. However, there are more complex issues associated with assessing treatment outcome that will be discussed later.

Necessary Measures for Time-Series Assessments in Stuttering Therapy

The next necessary assessment variable concerns the data measure(s). Just what should be measured? I believe there is now reasonable agreement that syllables spoken during talking time and stuttering frequency counts are necessary measures. They appear to be the bare minimum measures for determining changes in stuttering and the contribution that the amount and rate of speaking makes to stuttering variability.

All of us are sensitized to the notion that reduced speech rate may, in and of itself, reduce stuttering. Of course, reduced speaking as such may also have the same effect. Less publicized is the possibility that abnormally fast speech rate may also be associated with reduced stuttering (Ingham, Martin and Kuhl, 1974).

We are certainly not in agreement about how speech-rate should be measured. Ultimately, the speech-rate measurement issue boils down to contention about how it is to be measured, and what is a desirable or normally fluent speech rate. The issue of speed of speech, as Starkweather (1980) has recently pointed out, is much more complex than simple counts of words or syllables per minute. What is perceived as "fast" or "slow" turns out to be partially relative and also dependent upon variables such as sound durations, pause durations, coarticulation, and rate of syllable production. Consequently, our currently used clinical measures of rate provide only the sketchiest depiction of what is perceived as rate, or what might be normal rate. So, with this qualifier in mind, what options are available?

For some time some colleagues and I have used target rates of 170 to 210 syllables per minute as a guideline for normal rate (Ingham, 1981). But this measure is based on relatively unusual speech; a monologue that is not interrupted by the conversational exchanges that typify speech in the natural environment. Also, perhaps it is neither as useful nor as valid as Perkins' (1975) measure of articulation rate which excludes pauses. What, therefore, is an acceptable compromise? Whatever else, I believe that clinicians should be trained to count or rate syllables (and stutterings) on-line with the assistance of electronic button-press/counters that have been described in numerous research studies. These may be used as either articulation rate or syllable per minute counters. We actually have no data, at present, which indicate which measure more accurately reflects perceived speech rate. However, we do have some data from school children which indicate that the average syllables-per-minute rates in normal speech progressively increases over childhood. In the kindergarten years, for instance, the rate is around 50% of adult rates and rises to near adult rates by around 12 years (Kowal, O'Connor and Sabin, 1975). This might be used as a guide to estimate syllables-per-minute rates that should be achieved by the end of treatment. Perhaps a better alternative might be to take account of the child's speech rate during stutter-free intervals. And while these intervals may be influenced by the frequency of stutterings in the subject, at least they should give some idea of an acceptably normal rate for the speaker. Another useful guide might be the speech rates used by the child's peers: "normally fluent speech rate" may well be that which is used within the speaker's customary speaking environment. Finally, the clinician's perceptual judgment might be a useful guide, for there is no reason why a clinician's judgment of an acceptable and normal rate may not translate into clinically significant syllables-per-minute scores.

Clearly, stuttering counts are now accepted as another necessary measure. A frequency count of "moments of stuttering" may well be a less than perfect reflection of the quality of stuttering behavior. But it has certainly passed the test of time as a treatment measure, and probably for more reasons than the lassitude of clinicians and researchers. Some clinicians measure the length of stuttering intervals, or the disfluency categories of stutterings. But for therapy programs that are designed to remove all instances of stuttering, it is probably less important that those intervals be described as "severe" or "part-word repetitions"; the principal issue for most clinicians is whether stuttering continues to occur and how often it occurs over the number of syllables spoken by the subject. It also makes little sense to confound stuttering counts with counts of normal disfluencies. I think there is now general acceptance that clinicians (certainly lay observers) are able to distinguish between disfluencies and stutterings (MacDonald and Martin, 1973). This is an important consideration since there seems to be little obvious advantage in a treatment that succeeds in removing normal disfluencies, but fails to alter stutterings. Conversely, a treatment that aims to remove all disfluencies, normal or abnormal, may also run the risk of producing unusual sounding speech.

There are at least two dangers involved in relying upon frequency counts of stuttering alone as a measure for evaluating the performance of stutterers. The first relates to severity. Occasionally, a relatively low frequency of stuttering, certainly less than the much-touted 3% of words (Webster, 1979; Shine, 1980), may contain exceptionally long blocks. I am sure we all have encountered (Ingham, 1981) the very occasional subject who may produce less than 0.1% syllables stuttered, yet those stutterings may last for minutes. For this reason, there is obvious necessity in noting such unusual events. The second is a more troublesome issue—the role of word-avoidance. This must be the least researched stuttering phenomenon, yet it is also one of the best known. I am therefore uncertain as to whether it may influence stuttering frequency in children (it is not commonly associated with the speech behavior of young children). It is also not at all clear how it can be measured objectively. Perhaps the only control over its presence is the subject's report and instructional tests for its influence. The latter may be carried out by asking the subject to try to minimize stuttering for an interval, possibly by "avoiding stutterings," and then comparing this interval with another in which the reverse instruction applies.

There are numerous reasons why speech rate and stuttering frequency measures are inadequate assessments of speech performance in stuttering therapy, even though they are necessary measures. The most important concerns the imperfect relationship between zero stuttering at "normal" speech rate and normally fluent speech (Ingham, 1981; Perkins, 1981). This concern stems mainly from the increasing use of treatments that rely upon unusual speech patterns such as prolonged speech to procure "fluency." I certainly share with Adams (1982) and others their concern over our failure to provide a satisfactory description of normally fluent speech. The main issues have been explored in the previously-mentioned review by Starkweather (1980) who concluded that fluent speech "is the quality of speech that includes rapid and easy, as well as smooth production." (Starkweather, 1980, p. 195).* However, the combination of measurement operations needed to quantify that type of speaking is yet to be made available for clinical research, let alone clinician usage.

There is at least one reasonably satisfactory alternative procedure for identifying normal sounding fluency, that is, via perceptual analysis techniques. This involves either clinician ratings of normal quality (for example, Perkins, 1973a) or comparisons between speech samples made by normally fluent speakers and the subject (Ingham and Packman, 1978; Runyan and Adams, 1978, 1979). Both techniques have some obvious administrative and procedural limitations. Clinician ratings have uncertain reliability and interpretive value, especially since none of the present rating scales (Jones and Azrin, 1969; Perkins, 1973a; Turnbaugh and Guitar, 1981) has been extensively assessed for its reliability or validity in the context of clinic usage. Actually it is known from a study by Ingham and Packman (1978) that neither Jones and Azrin's nor Perkins' scale gives a measure of normalcy that clearly distinguishes between normal speakers' speech and post-treated speech of stutterers. On the other hand, perceptual analysis procedures, such as those used by Ingham and Packman (1978) and Runyan and Adams (1978; 1979), are not especially viable for regular clinical use at present. Their main difficulty is that they have not been investigated in order to identify factors among normally fluent speakers that may influence listener judgments. Not all normally fluent speakers sound normal; they may have accents, use colloquialisms, be from a wider age range than the stutterers, or whatever. These are only some of many variables that may need to be investigated in conjunction with this procedure in order to insure that they do not influence listener judgments. Perhaps one interesting alternative is to use the subject as his or her own control by obtaining samples of the subject's stutter-free speech for perceptual

---

*Starkweather also discusses this in the first chapter of this book.

comparisons. In other words, if the subject's pre-treatment stutter-free intervals are judged as normal sounding then they could be used for comparisons with the subject's own speech samples drawn from treatment and/or post-treatment intervals. By necessity this method would be restricted to subjects who had a reasonably low frequency of stuttering.

The areas of therapy evaluation where analyses of speech quality should be made is an interesting issue in and of itself. During the pre-treatment phase some researchers (for example, Adams, 1980) have suggested that diagnostic analyses of the subject's speech quality should be used to select the treatment procedure. I will return to consider this application shortly. However, such analyses have been mainly recommended during and after treatment in order to indicate whether the treatment has produced unusual or normal speech quality. Such information would certainly help describe performance. But, it is not at all clear what should be *done* with this information to aid the client. Quite obviously it can be used as a "baserate" for assessing the effects of various "add on" techniques designed to improve the normal sounding quality of the subject's speech. But at an operational level the available possibilities are relatively limited. They virtually amount to manipulations of speech rate and intensity plus instructions on prosody. Nevertheless there is almost no experimental evidence showing that these manipulations do, in fact, achieve a shift toward normal speech quality. The one interesting exception is Jones and Azrin's (1969) study on rhythmic stimulation which found that lengthening the duration of the stimulus signal increased listener ratings of naturalness—although unhappily these increases were confounded by increases in stuttering. It is very apparent therefore that much more research is needed before the role of perceptual analysis techniques in assessment can be clearly identified.*

In general, therefore, what I wish to recommend is that the measurement process should produce data that have a dual function; (1) provide a basis for establishing within—and beyond—clinic treatment effects, and (2) contribute to treatment operations. In other words, where possible, the measures chosen should do much more than passively chart the subject's progress through therapy. They should also permit decisions about the efficacy of therapy and, even more desirably, they may be used as treatment agents. It is this last function, it

---

*Since this paper was written there has been much interest in a speech naturalness rating scale developed by Martin, Haroldson and Triden (1984). Some preliminary investigations in this writer's and Martin's laboratories suggest that this scale may assist in assessing and improving speech naturalness.

seems to me, that has some interesting possibilities for transfer and maintenance of therapy effects. But before I discuss those final phases of the proposed assessment format, I want to return to the baserate phase and discuss the content of assessment strategies during that period.

Baserate Assessment Procedures

Possibly the most important assessment matter in the baserate phase concerns the procedures that will permit the clinician to decide whether a child is suitable for therapy. There is now reasonable consensus that certain forms of speech behavior are relevant for determining the likelihood that a child will develop into a chronic stutterer. Certain types and frequencies of disfluencies are expected events during speech development but the form, frequency, and variability of certain classes of disfluency probably differ among those young children who are identified as stutterers. Adams (1977) and Curlee (1980) have recently provided useful reviews of the pertinent literature in this area, and have outlined some reasonable guidelines to help distinguish the nonfluent child who is at risk. To paraphrase Adams, the child diagnosed as an "incipient stutterer" exhibits at least 10% of disfluent words that are characterized by part-word repetitions, audible silent prolongations, and broken words. The *schwa* vowel is perceived, and there is difficulty in starting and/ or sustaining voicing or air-flow which is evident at transitions from voiceless to voice sounds. These speech problems may also be accompanied by bodily movements, and the whole diagnosis should be supplemented by pertinent information from the parents and child. Essentially, the same recommendations are made by Curlee (1980) with the additional interesting suggestion that the child should be assessed under different speaking conditions. For, unlike normally disfluent children (Martin, Haroldson, and Kuhl, 1972a, b), the incipient stutterer's disfluencies tend to vary under different speaking conditions.

In the case of young children, there may also be some advantage in arranging for spectrographic analyses of disfluencies that parents label "stutterings." Some years ago Stromsta (1965) provided some provocative data which suggested that comparisons between disfluent and fluent tokens from young children served to distinguish between those who were stuttering 10 years later and those who were not. The data were based on observations as to whether or not the disfluencies showed "lack of formant transitions and/or abnormal terminations of phonation" (Stromsta, 1965, p. 317). Ten years later most of the children who displayed these features remained stuttering and those who did not were stutter-free. Unfortunately, the level of confidence we can have in these data is somewhat questionable since, as Curlee (1980) noted, the analysis criteria for the spectrograms were not adequately operationalized and it is not known which of these children received therapy during the following decade. Furthermore, the study still awaits the benefit of replication.

Curlee's (1980) recommendation that the child's speech be assessed under different conditions brings us back to the task of choosing speaking conditions that will identify variability, this time within the clinic. Some useful guidelines have been suggested by Ryan and Costello. Ryan (1974) has developed a "Stuttering Interview" which contains tasks suitable mainly for school-age stutterers. Costello (1981) has also provided a set of within-clinic procedures that can be employed to test for variability as well as gauge responsiveness to potential therapy procedures. Many of these within-clinic measures of variability have multiple advantages, especially if it can be shown that they correlate with counterpart beyond-clinic conditions. For example, repeated within-clinic assessments of the child speaking with "significant others" may match counterpart ratings of the child's speech with the same persons outside the clinic. The most obvious gain from this happy coincidence is the possibility of confining the treatment to the clinic rather than in beyond-clinic conditions with their attendant organizational difficulties. With young children, Ryan (1974) recommends a variety of tasks including monologues, oral-reading (if possible), telephone conversations, and conversations that incorporate questions. These seem to be particularly worthwhile tasks in view of the data that Ryan (1974) has provided that show very different frequencies of stuttering across these tasks.

From all the foregoing, what should be regarded as common and necessary? The most obvious contenders are conversational speech, monologues, and oral-reading since they are useful for assessment and treatment. Perhaps the main reason oral-reading is included is because of its utility in certain forms of therapy, otherwise it is strange that stuttering assessments have placed so much store on a task that is rarely performed in the natural environment (except occasionally in the school setting). Nevertheless, it does have the advantage of controlling for word avoidance. Clinician-client conversations, heavily laced with questions, and telephone conversations are obviously good choices. The latter is especially useful because of its viability for beyond-clinic treatment and assessment, particularly with older-age children. The ideal duration of each of these tasks is yet another "unknown," but in the context of demands on clinician time, perhaps each should be around three minutes.

Most of the current stuttering assessment systems place great emphasis on questionnaires. The purpose of these questionnaires is to highlight factors such as an abnormal health history, unusual reactions to speaking situations, the patterns of parent behavior and other considerations that are likely to be relevant to treatment. And all may serve a useful function. But I am not at all certain that most of this information cannot be gained during the course of an interview that simply overviews these areas of the subject's life. I am even less certain that any of the questionnaires currently recommended for clinicians contribute anything to treatment or evaluation that cannot be derived from suitably obtained speech performance data. I am prepared to be corrected but from my reading of the treatment literature I am unable to discern any evidence showing that responses on the available questionnaires have influenced the direction of a treatment program. If my observation is correct, then they have as much functional value as a description of the color of the child's hair. Perhaps the only exception to this dismissive note, as I will mention later, are post-treatment questionnaires that rate the subject's reaction to treatment (e.g., Webster, 1974).

Treatment Choice
Assessment Procedures

The final consideration in the initial assessment is the method by which a therapy is chosen. It seems to me that we still have virtually no research-based information that will help clinicians choose a treatment. From the perspective of behaviorially-oriented treatments, there is a growing literature that indicates some procedures may benefit children of all ages. It is not the purpose of this paper to review those treatments but it may be of some interest to review some of the reported decision-making processes for those treatments. Costello (1980, 1981) has suggested that the initial evaluation should include three brief tests to determine the modifiability of a child's stuttering; instructions to "talk as perfectly as possible" (Costello, 1980, p. 19) speaking in rhythm and using prolonged speech. The first of these obviously indicates the extent to which the child may modify stuttering under "demand" conditions. Presumably, this also provides an opportunity to discern the forms of speaking the child may adopt that could confound any therapy gains. The other two probes are also recommended to gain some notion of the child's responsiveness to potential therapy strategies. In most respects, this procedure resembles the suggestions made by Guitar and Peters (1980).

Another interesting approach is a strategy outlined by Riley and Riley (1979; 1983). They have devised a procedure for assessing children (3-11 years) in terms of four "neurologic" and five "traditional" components of stuttering. The neurologic being "attending disorders," "auditory-processing disorders," "sentence-formulation disorders" and "oral-motor disorders." The traditional components are "high self-expectations," "manipulative stuttering," "disruptive communication environment," "unrealistic parental expectations" and "abnormal parental need for the child to stutter." The child (and parents) are rated on each of these components and a treatment is then formulated to deal with each of the more problematic components. The general results of the treatments based on these components have been favorable according to data presented by the Rileys, but these data give no evidence that progress in treatment or outcome actually depends upon the inclusion of treatment procedures derived from these components. In other words, at best these pre-treatment tasks are little more than sensible suggestions. For there are no data that show they accurately (or even inaccurately) predict a child's responsiveness to these procedures in therapy.

Another interesting approach to the therapy choice issue is offered by Adams (1980). For example, with children who exhibit "problems in commencing and sustaining voicing or air flow" (Adams, 1980, p. 291) Adams recommends a variation of Perkins' (1973b) breath stream management technique. This may be supplemented by Ryan's (1974) GILCU procedure. If the child's stuttering is not characterized by difficulties in commencing and maintaining vocalization, then another option is that they may have "slowness and uncertainty in the operation of various aspects of the language encoding process (for example, word retrieval)" (Adams, 1980, p. 293). The GILCU procedure is also recommended for this type of case since it gives "the child more time to manage the control integrative aspects of communication" (Adams, 1980, p. 293). More recently, Adams and Runyan (1981) have provided more detailed recommendations that flow from evaluation of the acoustic signal. But the clinical merit of these recommendations also await data-based investigations.

In the absence of relevant data on the therapy decision making process there appears to be virtue in the suggestions offered by Costello, Guitar and Peters, Adams and the Rileys. The current treatment literature and some implications of the treatments that have been described therein, also provides some plausible guidelines (Costello, 1983). In the case of young children, there is every indication that the contingency management procedures may be of benefit and may not demand significant alterations in the child's manner of speech production. In effect, the response contingent punishment schedules that are suggested in the studies by Martin, Kuhl, and Haroldson (1972) and Reed and Godden (1977); or the GILCU procedures used in studies by Ryan (1974), Mowrer (1975) and Costello (1980) are useful starting points. So too might be the modeling strategies described by Johnson (1980) and Gregory and Hill (1980) for very young children, although I'd prefer to wait for data. These seem preferable initial interventions over those that require marked modifications in the speech pattern. In other words, the procedures described by Perkins (1973) or Webster (1979) might form a useful second stage intervention.

Dismantling Therapy and Time-Series Assessment

It may well be that a number of treatments are tried before a therapy strategy is found that will achieve within- and beyond-clinic treatment gains. That is, strategies that succeed in achieving establishment and transfer of treatment gains. It is therefore necessary for the assessment process to incorporate strategies that will indicate when the initial phase of treatment should be replaced by maintenance strategies.

I believe there is now general agreement that maintenance strategies are necessary components of the therapy process, although it is often difficult to believe that if we consider the slight amount of research they have attracted. There are some very limited data available that demonstrate the efficacy of the maintenance strategies currently used in therapy (Boberg, Howie and Woods, 1977; Boberg, 1981) but there is virtually nothing to help us in our search for assessment procedures for this phase. To some extent, that task has been eased by some useful data that suggest that when beyond-clinic generalization occurs in the treatment of preschool children, then unassisted maintenance will follow (Prins and Ingham, 1983). But I am sure

I can achieve agreement in claiming the evidence is not so persuasive in the case of older-age children. Nevertheless, in order to establish the necessity or otherwise of maintenance treatment, we should have the benefit of our mutually acceptable assessment format. The logical reference source is the continuation of the assessment format used in baserate and the initial treatment phase. In other words, the immediate post-treatment phase should be seen as a counterpart to the baserate phase. By this principle repeated assessments should continue for at least four weeks. This also provides a source for estimating the initial stability (or instability) of these gains.

The dismantling of the therapy process may also involve an integration of treatment and assessment procedures. One internally valid method of establishing when treatment should be withdrawn is to use a point or phase when assessment and therapy-controlled measures of speech performance begin to blend. Martin, Kuhl and Haroldson (1972) demonstrated this strategy in a comparison of the treatment and nontreatment setting performance by two preschool stutterers treated by contingency arrangements. Costello (1975) also used this technique to good effect during within-clinic conditions by comparing nontreatment and treatment intervals over contingency managed therapy sessions.

Another strategy that I have investigated in recent years (Ingham, 1980, 1981, 1982) is to systematically withdraw the regular assessment process contingent upon sustained performance criteria and compare the subject's performance with intermittent covert assessments. This is also an example of how the beyond- (or within-) clinic assessment procedures might serve dual functions, that is, decrease the contact frequency with the client while remaining a useful source of speech behavior control.

The method that I have been using to continue maintenance and evaluation actually serves to illustrate how maintenance and outcome evaluation strategies are able to be gradually integrated. The core procedure is for the subject to return to the clinic initially for two once-weekly assessments and if the target behavior (0% syllables stuttered at between 170 and 210 SPM) is maintained in all within- and beyond-clinic assessments, then the subject "earns" a two-week rest from assessments. If these two-week-apart assessments achieve the target behavior, then the subject earns a four-week "rest" from assessments. This systematic and performance-contingent withdrawal of assessment continues until two 32-week-apart assessments are passed successfully. If the subject fails on any assessment (that is, has one stuttering or departs from the target speech rate on any task), then the subject returns to the weekly assessments. In the most recent applications of this procedure (Ingham, 1982) it has been used in conjunction with a self-management techniques (specifically, self-evaluation training) in order to shift the responsibility for conducting this performance-contingent assessment strategy to the subject. In the main, these procedures have been used with a good measure of success with adults, but they have also been found effective with older-age children (Ingham, 1980). The data from these studies have been supplemented by nonperformance-contingent assessments made in beyond-clinic conditions, which thereby serve to establish the point when the non-treatment related assessments blend with the treatment assessments. They have also been supplemented by a wide variety of covert assessments that have shown, in some cases, that overt assessments certainly do not equate with the covert assessments. To a large extent, though, these concurrent assessments have suggested that the maintenance strategy may be phased-out well before the 32-week-apart assessment point.

Undoubtedly, covert assessment procedures are among the most contentious assessment techniques used in stuttering therapy. But in their defense, I would contend that they have the potential of providing the most clinically-valid treatment assessment data, particularly when used in conjunction with relevant overt assessment data. Their claim to validity, however, is only as strong as their claims to be unobtrusive—and these claims are often difficult to demonstrate. There are various degrees of "covertness," or varieties of techniques that might be free of some of the reactive features found in overt assessments. Features that many clinicians suspect produce unrealistic or "artificial" post-treatment data. Perhaps the most useful of these is the "unplanned telephone call," made ideally by a person not associated with the treatment. Other relevant information may be derived from parents or friends of the subject, which can then be validated by suitably arranged recordings. Admittedly, this all sounds uncomfortably unethical, but it need not be. In the case of older-age children, it is unlikely that the validity of this form of assessment will be threatened if, before treatment, the client agrees that such assessments will be made from time to time in order to test the worth of treatment. I have used this procedure on numerous occasions over the past decade, and I have yet to meet one client who found it to be distasteful or disconcerting. More importantly, it has often provided an immensely useful clinical service. For instance, in the current applications of the maintenance schedule described above, my clinicians intermittently telephone subjects. If they detect a stuttering then, regardless of whether the subject "passed" the previous assessment, the subject automatically fails that assessment and returns to the initial step in the maintenance schedule.

How should covert assessment be organized within an assessment schedule? Like all other assessment decisions, I believe that the method should be guided, where possible, by treatment and evaluation considerations. However, the difficulty with this form of assessment is that it may lose its validity if it is used too frequently, and quite obviously, if the subject becomes aware of its occurrence. At the very least, it seems to me, that this type of assessment carries treatment and assessment value if it occurs once during the transfer phase of treatment and again during the immediate post-treatment assessment phase. This allows the clinician to decide whether the subject's assessed speech performance is indeed reflected in less stimulus-bound conditions. Probably, the most practical procedure for this purpose, is an unannounced telephone conversation with a person unconnected with the treatment. It is up to the clinician to decide how this should be recorded, but there is no reason why it cannot be rated on-line by a trained clinician. The frequency with which covert assessments should be made during the maintenance phase largely depends on the duration of that phase. Of course, in turn, this raises the issue of time spans for post-treatment assessments, the final phase of our format.

Follow-Up Assessment

In the case of child or adult therapy, our literature has little to offer as justification for prescribed follow-up intervals or assessments. The typical recommendations are that post-treatment assessments should occur at intervals ranging from a few weeks to five years (Silverman, 1981). What this reflects is yet another area of confusion, this time about the function of post-treatment evaluation. The primary purpose of follow-up evaluation is surely to establish whether the child is unimproved, improved, or free of his problem after a period in which variables likely to influence the problem have had every opportunity to occur. The difficulty is that we have very little idea about the nature of these variables. But the fact that a child has improved or not improved speech performance at follow-up may have very little to do with treatment. Quite clearly, the longer the interval between cessation of treatment and follow-up evaluation, the more likely it is that this interval will be filled with variables of far more relevance to current performance than the original treatment. I hasten to add that we also have little idea about the nature of these variables. But there are some logical contenders; practice regimes, "significant other" control of speech performance, and even additional treatment are good prospects for consideration.

At best, I believe that follow-up evaluation may give the clinician and client knowledge about the current state of the disorder and some useful hypotheses about the durability of the treatment's effects. For this reason, it seems that the most practical guideline for follow-up evaluation is to schedule assessments over the following year. At least this accommodates to annual timetabling arrangements, and is consistent with the intervals used in many clinical studies.

The frequency of follow-up assessments presents another imponderable. Perhaps the logical solution is to use the "four-data-point" principle from our therapy assessment format. This means that follow-up assessments should occur at three-month intervals. And in order to determine the validity of this trend, perhaps these assessments should be interspersed with another four covert assessments.

The content of these post-treatment assessments warrants a few additional comments. The logical contenders are the within- and beyond-clinic assessments used over the initial therapy phases. Perhaps the most practical option for covert assessment is a three-to-five minute surprise telephone call involving a question-answer conversation with a stranger. But at least two other assessments are important; the perceptual analysis assessment of the subject's speech quality and a questionnaire similar to that devised by Webster (1974). A copy of this questionnaire is in Appendix 2 at the end of this chapter. For my money the main value of this questionnaire is that it solicits the subjects' judgement on the extent to which he must attend to his speech in order to continue to speak fluently. At present, I know of no other means of determining the extent to which therapy gains are sustained at the cost of unusual levels of attention to speaking. Once again, there are no available norms on this form of questionnaire—indeed, I am not sure how these could be interpreted—but it might be expected that over the follow-up period there should be some evidence that the subject's level of attention to his speech declines in concert with sustained improvements. That would seem to be one of the more clinically valid indicators of treatment success.

Conclusions

Let us now try to put together all the pieces of our therapy assessment puzzle. It begins with a series of diagnostic sessions designed to establish the child's suitability for therapy. This is followed by a baserate period containing repeated within- and beyond-clinic recorded assessments conducted twice-weekly over at least four weeks. They continue at this frequency throughout the establishment and transfer phases of therapy, and for at least four more weeks into the maintenance phase. The maintenance phase may include decreasingly frequent assessments that might also be tied to the treatment process. The pattern of maintenance assessment should continue until they occur at three-month intervals. At this point, they should fade into follow-up assessments made at three-month intervals over a year. The overt assessment procedure should be supplemented by at least one covert assessment during treatment and another during the four-week immediate post-treatment phase. In addition, perhaps covert assessments, of one form or another, should be made at regular intervals over the maintenance and follow-up periods. The content of the overt assessments should include representative speech samples from the speaker's natural environment plus oral-readings, monologues and telephone conversations within the clinic. The minimum data collected should be syllable or articulation rate and percentage of words or syllables stuttered. These data should be supplemented by perceptual analyses or ratings of speech quality. Finally, the post-treatment phase of therapy should be supplemented by a questionnaire reporting the subject's estimate of his or her speech performance.

Quite obviously, this is an unrealistic format for very young children—indeed it is probably suitable mainly for the seven to 12-year-old age group. However, it should be equally obvious that those components that are not suitable for young children can be removed or modified without too much threat to their viability. For example, parent recordings may replace subject-collected recordings, and the duration of post-treatment assessments may be reduced. At the same time, I believe that substantial amounts of this format can be used with young children. That has certainly been the case in my association with the treatments for this age group.

I would like to end my presentation with a plea. I wish to plead that this format be given serious consideration as one means of shifting stuttering therapy towards a reasonably common assessment format which makes it possible to develop knowledge about the therapy process—knowledge that will be of immense benefit to all concerned with this disorder. There is an almost desperate need for a data-base from field clinicians on current stuttering therapy procedures. If clinicians could be encouraged to gather and report data within the format that I have described, then I feel certain that we would be considerably advanced in solving that need. For only clinicians can show the strengths and weaknesses of these treatments in the field rather than in the research "laboratory."

TREATMENT EFFECT SURVEY

This table summarizes the results of a survey of stuttering treatments involving children 12 years of age or younger. The survey was designed to identify studies in which it was possible to discern the treatment time needed for individual subjects to reduce stuttering or disfluencies by more than 50% relative to baserate. That point was established when the target behavior reached the 50% reduction level on two assessment occasions. In the case of the "Gradual Increase in Length and Complexity of Utterance" (GILCU) and speech pattern treatments, the 50% reduction level was regarded as equivalent to half the time required to achieve the study's designated treatment target.

Method	Procedure	Study	Time required to reach 50% reduction in target behavior relative to B/R (hours)	Age
Response Contingent	GILCU	Costello (1980)	15.50	11
		Johnson et al (1978)	10.50	6
		Ryan (1974)	10.45	7
		Ryan (1974)	30.05	7
		Ryan (1974)	4.85	8
		Ryan (1974)	3.30	8
		Ryan (1974)	7.70	9
		Ryan (1974)	12.65	8
Response Contingent	Positive Reinforcement	Peters (1977)	0.60	8
		Peters (1977)	0.60	8
		Shaw and Shrum (1972)	0.67	9
		Shaw and Shrum (1972)	0.67	9
		Shaw and Shrum (1972)	0.67	10
Response Contingent	Combined Punishment and Reinforcement	Ryan (1974)	1.00	9
		Ryan (1974)	6.00	9
Response Contingent	Punishment	Martin and Berndt (1970)	0.67	12
		Martin et al (1972)	1.33	3
		Martin et al (1972)	2.00	4
		McDermott (1971)	1.20	9
		Reed and Godden (1977)	1.33	5
		Reed and Godden (1977)	1.67	3

Method	Procedure	Study	Time required to reach 50% reduction in target behavior relative to B/R (hours)	Age
Speech Pattern	Prolonged Speech	Ryan (1971)	2.00	8
		Ryan (1974)	5.65	8
		Ryan (1974)	20.25	12
		Turnbaugh and Guitar (1981)	4.50	12
Speech Pattern	Regulated Breathing	Azrin and Nunn (1974)	1.00	4
		Azrin and Nunn (1974)	1.00	9
		Hee and Holmes (1976)	1.50	10
Speech Pattern	Shadowing	Ottoni (1974)	1.00	9
Traditional	Programmed	Ryan (1974)	2.30	10

appendix two
CLIENTS' SELF-RATING ON FOLLOW-UP QUESTIONNAIRE*

1. Rate your current overall level of fluency.
   - ☐ Essentially fluent speech
     (None, or very few, hard sounds. No Noticeable repetitions.)
   - ☐ Good fluency
     (A few hard sounds: some small hesitations, a few repetitions.)
   - ☐ Adequate fluency
     (Quite a few hard sounds. A good many short hesitations and/or repetitions. Some, but not much, stuttering occurred.)
   - ☐ Marginal fluency
     (Many hard sounds. A lot of hesitations and/or repetitions. Quite a bit of stuttering, but not as much as before fluency shaping.)
   - ☐ Disfluent speech
     (Stuttering at about the same frequency and duration as before fluency shaping.)

2. Was the Precision Fluency Shaping Program worthwhile for you?
   - ☐ Very much
   - ☐ Quite a bit
   - ☐ A moderate amount
   - ☐ A small amount
   - ☐ Of no benefit

3. How satisfied were you with your speech fluency before the Precision Fluency Shaping Program?
   - ☐ Very satisfied
   - ☐ Satisfied
   - ☐ Neither satisfied nor unsatisfied
   - ☐ Unsatisfied
   - ☐ Very unsatisfied

4. How satisfied were you with your speech fluency immediately after the Precision Fluency Shaping Program?
   - ☐ Very satisfied
   - ☐ Satisfied
   - ☐ Neither satisfied nor unsatisfied
   - ☐ Unsatisfied
   - ☐ Very unsatisfied

5. How satisfied are you with your present speech fluency?
   - ☐ Very satisfied
   - ☐ Satisfied
   - ☐ Neither satisfied nor unsatisfied
   - ☐ Unsatisfied
   - ☐ Very unsatisfied

---

*from Webster, R. L., *The Precision Fluency Shaping Program: Speech Reconstruction for Stutterers*, Roanoke, Virginia: Hollins Communication Research Institute, 1974.

6. Is your present speech fluency improved over the quality of your speech before coming to Hollins?
   ☐ Very much improved
   ☐ Substantially improved
   ☐ Moderately improved
   ☐ Slightly improved
   ☐ No improved

7. How much attention must you pay to the task of speaking fluently?
   ☐ Less than 1/10 of daily speech situations
   ☐ Less than 1/3 of daily speech situations
   ☐ From 1/3 to 2/3 of daily speech situations
   ☐ More than 2/3 of daily speech situations
   ☐ Attention required in all speech situations

8. Have you had any other stuttering therapy since leaving the Precision Fluency Shaping Program?
   ☐ Yes
   ☐ No

9. Do you have more confidence in your speech now than you did before entering the Precision Fluency Shaping Program?
   ☐ Yes
   ☐ No
   ☐ Undecided

10. Do you have more confidence in yourself now?
   ☐ Yes
   ☐ No
   ☐ Undecided

References

Adams, M. R., "A Clinical Strategy for Differentiating the Normally Nonfluent Child and the Incipient Stutterer," *Journal of Fluency Disorders*, 2, 141-148, 1977.

Adams, M. R., "The Young Stutterer: Diagnosis, Treatment and Assessment of Progress," *Seminars in Speech, Language and Hearing*, 1, 289-299, 1980.

Adams, M. R., "Fluency, Nonfluency, and Stuttering in Children," *Journal of Fluency Disorders*, 7, 171-185, 1982.

Adams, M. R., and Runyan, C. M., "Stuttering and Fluency: Exclusive Events or Points on a Continuum?" *Journal of Fluency Disorders*, 6, 197-218, 1981.

Andrews, G., and Harvey, R., "Regression to the Mean in Pretreatment Measures of Stuttering," *Journal of Speech and Hearing Disorders*, 46, 204-207, 1981.

Azrin, N. H., and Nunn, R. G., "A Rapid Method of Eliminating Stuttering by a Regulated Breathing Approach," *Behaviour Research and Therapy*, 12, 279-286, 1974.

Birnbrauer, J. S., "External Validity and Experimental Investigation of Individual Behaviour," *Analysis and Intervention in Developmental Disabilities*, 1, 117-132, 1981.

Boberg, E. (Ed.), *Maintenance of Fluency*. New York: Elsevier, 1981.

Boberg, E., Howie, P., and Woods, L., "Maintenance of Fluency: A Review," *Journal of Fluency Disorders*, 4, 93-116, 1979.

Costello, J. M., "The Establishment of Fluency with Time-out Procedures: Three Case Studies," *Journal of Speech and Hearing Disorders*, 40, 216-231, 1975.

Costello, J. M., "Operant Conditioning and the Treatment of Stuttering," *Seminars in Speech, Language and Hearing*, 1, 311-327, 1980.

Costello, J. M., "Pretreatment Assessment of Stuttering in Young Children," *Communicative Disorders: An Audio Journal for Continuing Education*. New York: Grune and Stratton, 1981.

Costello, J. M., "Current Behavioral Treatments for Children," in Prins, D., and Ingham, R. J. (Eds.), *Treatment of Stuttering in Early Childhood: Methods and Issues*. San Diego: College-Hill Press, In press, 1983.

Curlee, R. F., "A Case Selection Strategy for Young Disfluent Children," *Seminars in Speech, Language and Hearing*, 1, 277-287, 1980.

Gregory, H. H., and Hill, D., "Stuttering Therapy for Children," *Seminars in Speech, Language and Hearing*, 1, 351-363, 1980.

Guitar, B., and Peters, A. D., *Stuttering: An Integration of Contemporary Therapies*. Memphis: Speech Foundation of America, 1980.

Hee, J. C., and Holmes, P. A., "Elimination of Stuttering by a Regulated Breathing Approach," *Journal of Communication Pathology*, 8, 40-44, 1976.

Hersen, M., and Barlow, D. H., *Single Case Experimental Designs: Strategies for Studying Behavior Change*. New York: Pergamon Press, 1976.

Ingham, R. J., "Modification of Maintenance and Generalization During Stuttering Treatment," *Journal of Speech and Hearing Research*, 23, 732-745, 1980.

Ingham, R. J., "Evaluation and Maintenance in Stuttering Treatment: A Search for Ecstasy with Nothing But Agony," in Boberg, E. (Ed.), *Main-

tenance of Fluency. New York: Elsevier, 1981.

Ingham, R. J., "The Effects of Self-Evaluation Training on Maintenance and Generalization During Stuttering Treatment," *Journal of Speech and Hearing Disorders,* In press, 1982.

Ingham, R. J., and Lewis, J. I., "Behavior Therapy and Stuttering: And the Story Grows," *Human Communication,* 3, 125-152, 1978.

Ingham, R. J., and Packman, A., "Treatment and Generalization Effects in an Experimental Treatment for a Stutterer Using Contingency Management and Speech Rate Control," *Journal of Speech and Hearing Disorders,* 42, 394-407, 1977.

Ingham, R. J., and Packman, A. C., "Perceptual Assessment of Normalcy of Speech Following Stuttering Therapy," *Journal of Speech and Hearing Research,* 21, 63-73, 1978.

Johnson, G. F., Coleman, K., and Rasmussen, K., "Multidays: Multidimensional Approach for the Young Stutterer," *Language, Speech and Hearing Services in Schools,* 9, 129-132, 1978.

Johnson, L. J., "Facilitating Parental Involvement in Therapy of the Disfluent Child," *Seminars in Speech, Language and Hearing,* 1, 301-309, 1980.

Jones, R. J., and Azrin, N. H., "Behavioral Engineering: Stuttering as a Function of Stimulus Duration During Speech Synchronization," *Journal of Applied Behavior Analysis,* 2, 223-229, 1969.

Kowal, S., O'Connell, D. C., and Sabin, E. F., "Development of Temporal Patterning and Vocal Hesitations in Spontaneous Narratives," *Journal of Psycholinguistic Research,* 4, 195-207, 1975.

MacDonald, J. D., and Martin, R. R., "Stuttering and Disfluency as Two Reliable and Unambiguous Response Classes," *Journal of Speech and Hearing Research,* 16, 691-699, 1973.

Martin, R. R., and Berndt, L. A., "The Effects of Time-out on Stuttering in a 12 Year Old Boy," *Exceptional Children,* 36, 303-304, 1970.

Martin, R. R., Haroldson, S. K., and Kuhl, P., "Disfluencies in Childchild and Child-mother Speaking Situations," *Journal of Speech and Hearing Research,* 15, 753-756, 1972a.

Martin, R. R., Haroldson, S. K., and Kuhl, P., "Disfluencies of Young Children in Two Speaking Situations," *Journal of Speech and Hearing Research,* 15, 831-836, 1972b.

Martin, R. R., Haroldson, S. K., and Triden, K. A., "Stuttering and Speech Naturalness," *Journal of Speech and Hearing Disorders,* 49, 53-58, 1984.

Martin, R. R., Kuhl, P., and Haroldson, S. K., "An Experimental Treatment with Two Preschool Stuttering Children," *Journal of Speech and Hearing Research,* 15, 743-752, 1972.

McDermott, L. D., "Clinical Management of Stuttering Behavior: A Case Study," *Feedback,* 1, 6-7, 1971.

Mowrer, D., "An Instructional Program to Increase Fluent Speech of Stutterers," *Journal of Fluency Disorders,* 1, 25-35, 1975.

Ottoni, T. M., "Uso de la tecnica delineamento del habla para cambiar la conducta verbal," *Revista Interamericana de Psicologia,* 8, 3-4, 1974.

Perkins, W. H., *Behavioral Management of Stuttering.* Final report. Social and Rehabilitation Service Research Grant 14-P-55281, University of Southern California, 1973a.

Perkins, W. H., "Replacement of Stuttering with Normal Speech. II. Clinical Procedures," *Journal of Speech and Hearing Disorders,* 38, 295-303, 1973b.

Perkins, W. H., "Articulatory Rate in the Evaluation of Stuttering Treatments," *Journal of Speech and Hearing Disorders*, 40, 277-278, 1975.

Perkins, W. H., "Measurement and Maintenance of Fluency," in Boberg, E. (Ed.), *Maintenance of Fluency*. New York: Elsevier, 1981.

Peters, A. D., "The Effect of Positive Reinforcement on Fluency: Two Case Studies," *Language, Speech and Hearing Services in Schools*, 8, 15-22, 1977.

Prins, D., and Ingham, R. J., *Treatment of Stuttering in Early Childhood: Methods and Issues*. San Diego: College-Hill Press, In press, 1983.

Reed, C. G., and Godden, A. L., "An Experimental Treatment Using Verbal Punishment with Two Preschool Stutterers," *Journal of Fluency Disorders*, 2, 225-233, 1977.

Riley, G., and Riley, J., "A Component Model for Diagnosing and Treating Children Who Stutter," *Journal of Fluency Disorders*, 4, 279-294, 1979.

Riley, G., and Riley, J., "Evaluation as a Basis for Intervention," in Prins, D., and Ingham, R. J. (Eds.), *Treatment of Stuttering in Early Childhood: Methods and Issues*. San Diego: College-Hill Press, In press, 1983.

Runyan, C. M., and Adams, M. R., "Perceptual Study of the Speech of 'Successfully Therapeutized' Stutterers," *Journal of Fluency Disorders*, 3, 25-39, 1978.

Runyan, C. M., and Adams, M. R., "Unsophisticated Judges' Perceptual Evaluations of the Speech of 'Successfully Treated' Stutterers," *Journal of Fluency Disorders*, 4, 29-38, 1979.

Ryan, B. P., "Operant Procedures Applied to Stuttering Therapy for Children," *Journal of Speech and Hearing Disorders*, 36, 264-280, 1971.

Ryan, B. P., *Programmed Therapy for Stuttering in Children and Adults*. Springfield, Illinois: C. C. Thomas, 1974.

Shaw, C. K., and Shrum, W. F., "The effects of Response-contingent Reward on the Connected Speech of Children Who Stutter," *Journal of Speech and Hearing Disorders*, 37, 75-88, 1972.

Shine, R. E., "Direct Management of the Beginning Stutterer," *Seminars in Speech, Language and Hearing*, 1, 339-350, 1980.

Silverman, F. H., "Relapse Following Stuttering Therapy," in Lass, N. J. (Ed.), *Speech and Language: Advances in Basic Research and Practice*, Volume 5. New York: Academic Press, 1981.

Starkweather, C. W., "Speech Fluency and Its Development in Normal Children," in Lass, N. J. (Ed.), *Speech and Language: Advances in Basic Research and Practice*, Volume 4. New York: Academic Press, 1980.

Stromsta, C., "A Spectrographic Study of Dysfluencies Labeled as Stuttering by Parents," *De Therapia Vocis et Loquelae (Proceedings XIII International Congress of Logopedics and Phoniatrics, Vienna)*, Volume 1, 317-319, 1965.

Turnbaugh, K. R., and Guitar, B. E., "Short-term Intensive Stuttering Treatment in a Public School Setting," *Language, Speech and Hearing Services in Schools*, 12, 107-114, 1981.

Webster, R. L., *The Precision Fluency Shaping Program: Speech Reconstruction for Stutterers*. Roanoke, Virginia: Hollins Communications Research Institute, 1974.

Webster, R. L., "Empirical Considerations Regarding Stuttering Therapy," in Gregory, H. H. (Ed.), *Controversies About Stuttering Therapy*. Baltimore: University Park Press, 1979.

chapter six

Integration: Present Status and Prospects for the Future

Hugo H. Gregory, Ph.D.
Northwestern University

When to be Concerned About a Child's Fluency

Parents will say, "I think my child is beginning to stutter," or "He has been stuttering for several months," or "Is Johnny stuttering?" Speech and language pathologists are then called upon to listen to the child's speech, describe disfluencies, render a judgment, and give an opinion. In sampling the child's speech, the clinician must take into consideration the influence of situational factors and such language factors as meaningfulness and length of utterance as described by Hanley, Nelson, and Williams.* Obviously, defining the existence of a stuttering problem with reference to the appropriate observation of a child's speech is a rather complex matter and far from being an "either or" matter.

---

*In this chapter, when no bibliographic date is given, the reference is to the author's chapter in this book. Page numbers accompanying quotes with no date of reference refer to page numbers in this volume.

In chapter 4, Starkweather refers at length to Kowal, O'Connell, and Sabin's study (1975) of disfluencies in kindergarten through twelfth grade students. When all disfluencies are considered, the amount of total disfluency does not change much during this period (all children are disfluent), but the type of disfluency does. In this age range, part-word repetitions decline sharply between kindergarten or first grade and the fourth grade, and false starts decline, especially between the 4th and 6th grades. Thus, Starkweather states that a fourth grader with a high frequency of part-word repetition might be said to be immature in this respect.

In general, part word sound and syllable repetitions and prolongations of sounds have been found to be the least frequently occurring disfluencies in the speech of pre-school children (Brownell, 1973; De Joy, 1975; Haynes and Hood, 1977; Wexler and Mysak, 1982). Data from Johnson (1955) and Yairi (1981) indicate that two year olds may show considerable part-word repetition, but most studies indicate that part-word repetition begins to decrease during the third year (Johnson, 1955; Yairi, 1982). Single syllable word repetitions are fairly frequent in a child's speech during the second or third years when relational language is developing rapidly.

The rather large intersubject and intrasubject variability (the latter based on repeated measures of disfluency types in the same child taken at 3 or 4 month intervals) is another complicating factor in our assessment of disfluency in a child's speech. Yairi (1982) concludes:

> Unlike several other aspects of speech and language such as sound acquisition, articulatory precision, and syntactic skills that usually assume a one-way developmental course, disfluency stands out as a phenomenon which is prone to alternating reversals. (p. 159)

This observation probably reflects the possibility that many factors influence fluency, a notion with considerable common sense appeal and again one that makes our evaluation process difficult. This also complicates definitive research.

What can we conclude from our present information?

(1) Pauses, revisions, and interjections (non-repetitious disfluencies) occur most frequently in the speech of pre-school children.

(2) One syllable word repetitions occur rather frequently in the speech of most children.

(3) Breaks in fluency at the word level (sound and syllable repetitions and prolongations of sounds) occur less

frequently in the speech of most children. Therefore, we are more concerned about increases of these disfluency types in a child's speech.

(4) We are more concerned about one syllable word repetitions or part-word repetition if there is a high frequency of repetition per instance—4 or more with relatively even rhythm and stress and 2 or more with relatively uneven rhythm and stress (Gregory and Hill, 1980).

(5) Concern is greater if there is a disruption of air flow or phonation between repetitions or if a schwa sounding vowel is substituted for the one ordinarily used in the repetition of a syllable (Cooper, 1973; Adams, 1977; Curlee, 1980; Gregory and Hill, 1980; VanRiper, 1982).

(6) Other signs of increased tension in the lips, jaw, larynx, or chest are more obvious characteristics that create more concern and point more definitely to a problem.

These statements reflect a continuum of disfluent speech behaviors from *More Usual* to *More Unusual* that Hill and I have published in 1980 (see Figure 1). We like the continuum idea because it reflects our present knowledge about children's disfluency and we are comfortable with the use of concern in describing our evaluation because it lends itself to the consideration of degree.

In conclusion, it seems that we have made considerable progress in understanding the types of disfluency that occur with greater or lesser frequency in the speech of children, the variable nature of disfluency in children, and the aspects of part-word repetition and one syllable word repetition that signal more unusual fragmentation and disruption of the vocal tract dynamics of speech production. Distortions in a child's speech flow such as general tension, tense glottal strokes, etc., not just the moment of disfluency or stuttering, are important to note and to consider in therapy. We should follow Costello's advice (Costello, 1980) to describe each child's speech carefully to record unique behavior demonstrated.

Conference participants expressed the belief that studies of speech fluency in children (Johnson, 1955; Brownell, 1973; Haynes and Hood, 1977; Wexler and Mysak, 1982; Yairi, 1981, 1982) and carefully reported clinical observations (Cooper, 1973; Adams, 1977; Curlee, 1980; Gregory and Hill, 1980; VanRiper, 1982) should enable practicing clinicians to put together a speech analysis procedure that makes it possible for them to be fairly objective and to have confidence in their decisions. As mentioned previously, and as emphasized by Ingham, we are dealing with

FIGURE 1

Continuum of Disfluent Speech Behaviors

More Usual

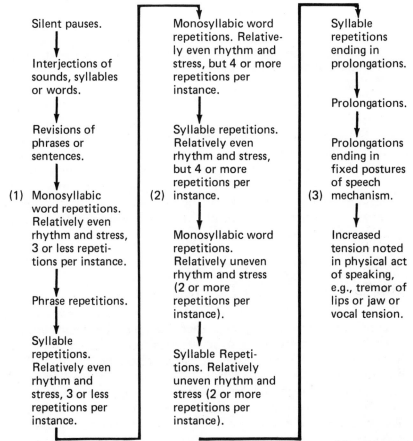

More Unusual

(1) Typical disfluencies that occur in pre-school children's speech. Listed on the continuum in general order of expected frequency (silent pauses the most frequent).

(2) Borderline atypical disfluencies that occur less frequently in the speech of children. For frame of reference, in a speech sample of 500 words or more, if there are 2 or more of any one of these behaviors per 100 words, this should be considered a basis for concern and especially so if air flow or phonation is disrupted between the repetitions or if a schwa sounding vowel is substituted for the one ordinarily used in the repetition of a syllable (for example, "Mə Mə Mə Ma Ma"). May be referred to as "cross-over behaviors" on the continuum between "more usual" and "more unusual" speech disfluencies.

(3) Atypical disfluencies that are very infrequent in the speech of children.

(Continued on next page)

FIGURE 1

Continuum of Disfluent Speech Behaviors
(Continued from page 133)

More characteristic of what listeners perceive as stuttering. If 1 or more prolongations occur per 100 words in a speech sample of 500 words or more, this should be considered a basis for considerable concern. Of course, fixed postures or other signs of increased tension and fragmentation of the flow of speech should be a basis for immediate attention.

(From Gregory and Hill, 1980)

behavior that shows considerable variability; therefore, this should be kept in mind. One observation of a child is not sufficient. In addition, when we choose an intervention strategy, we should monitor the child's disfluency at home and in other situations such as nursery school, as well as at the clinic, in order to check the ongoing nature of the child's speech development.

A Broader View of Fluency — Disfluency Versus Discontinuity

Starkweather emphasizes that there is more to be looked at in considering the fluency of speech than just the *discontinuities* in speech production such as pauses, hesitations, and repetitions. In his view, a measure of fluency should also take into consideration rate and ease of production. Therefore, what we commonly term disfluencies should be designated as discontinuities. When we look at it this way, continuity is only one aspect of fluency. Starkweather states that we need better information about the development of continuity, rate, speech effort, and rhythm. He points to the need for large sample studies of these characteristics in pre-school children.

Participants in the conference were especially intrigued by Starkweather's point that many of the discontinuities that we now call disfluencies such as pauses, interjections, revisions, even word repetitions, may be corrections that *contribute to increased fluency* in the child's speech. He states: "The odd thing about these discontinuities is the persistent belief that people seem to have that they are errors of speech" (p. 18). Starkweather concludes that part-word repetitions do not appear to serve a correcting function nor do prolongations. One may take this as additional evidence that sound and syllable repetitions and prolongations are more unusual, and possibly more pathological disfluencies depending on certain quantitative and qualitative characteristics. Finally, Starkweather's presentations prompted considerable discussion of the possibility that spectographic analysis of repetitious disfluencies (discontinuities according to Starkweather) may reveal characteristics that will enable us to identify vocal tract functions that are more "deviant" in some children. Research now underway at Syracuse University as well as other centers may enhance our knowledge of the way in which our perceptions of fluency and disfluency are related to acoustic analysis and simultaneous physiological events at the levels of respiration, phonation, and articulation.

Starkweather's discussion of fluency reminds us that in terms of intervention, the clinician's goal should be for the child to have speech that is not just smooth, as contrasted to fragmented, but also within normal range in rate, inflection, and ease of production. Of course, both Starkweather and Ingham reminded us that it is sometimes difficult to say what is normal since there is so much variation. Oftentimes, children who have been through stuttering therapy seem to me to have better speech than some of their peers. Slower speech may be acceptable as a stage in therapy, but therapy should not be terminated until speech is within the normal range in all respects. In our own work with children, we keep the distortions in rate and prosody, which may be necessary at first to get a smooth flow, at a minimum. In summary, the range of normal is rather broad, but we do not want therapy to result in speech that is smoother, yet calls attention to itself because prosody and rate are distinctive.

Factors Related to Increased Disfluency and Stuttering

The Conference Planning Committee decided that environmental, motoric, and linguistic factors should be examined carefully. This decision was related to the amount of research that has been done, our clinical knowledge of the factors that influence the variability of disfluency and stuttering, and the renewed interest during the last ten years in linguistic and motoric aspects of stuttering (St. Louis, 1979; Starkweather, 1982). The big questions we wanted to ask were: What meaning can the clinician devoted to the prevention of stuttering and early intervention with the beginning stutterer make out of the knowledge available? The children who need help are a present reality. What do we do for these children and their parents or their teachers?

Finally, what developments presently underway hold promise for the future?

During discussions, following the lectures presented as chapters in this book, participants kept several "facts" in mind as basic and agreed upon. The vast majority of stuttering begins in childhood, most between 30 months and 60 months, but we often say between ages 2 to 7 years of age since some cases are reported as beginning when the child starts to school. There appears to be a genetic factor that predisposes certain children to stuttering, but environmental factors are assumed to interact with these genetic dispositions. The male-female ratio is probably 3 or 4 to 1. About 2/3 of children who show a noticable degree of stuttering at sometime during their development, regain normal fluency ("recover from stuttering"). This last observation is based on retrospective research, clinical observations, and parent reports.

Nelson reviewed the literature relating the occurrence of disfluency to language factors showing that disfluency in non-stuttering and stuttering children does show some interesting relationships to the initiation of syntactic units, the complexity of syntactic transformations and the child's syntactic maturity. Nelson referred to fairly recent journal reports (Hall, 1977; Merits-Patteson and Reed, 1981) that have offered better evidence for the observation, made by most clinicians, that as children in language therapy develop improved syntax and vocabulary, they often have episodes of excessive disfluency. A survey (Blood and Seider, 1981) has shown that children who stutter tend to have a high incidence of problems of articulation and language. This agrees with data that has been reported over a period of decades indicating that stuttering children are late in passing language developmental milestones and have a higher incidence of articulation problems. More and more, clinicians are accepting the assumption that some beginning stuttering children have concomitant articulation and language problems of clinical significance, or of a minimal nature, that may contribute to increased disfluency (or stuttering), or may be important in maintaining stuttering.

Although there are some contradictory research findings, adult stutterers show signs of minimal auditory processing problems based on the use of such procedures as dichotic listening employing meaningful linguistic stimuli (Curry and Gregory, 1969; Sommers, Brady, and Moore, 1975; Quinn, 1972) and auditory test batteries (Hall and Jerger, 1978; Toscher and Rupp, 1978). The auditory system of children needs to be studied more. With patience and care, evoked response audiometry can be used with children, and since this does not involve a behavioral response, this procedure may be used to provide more information about the auditory system and stuttering.* The clinician will, of course, ask, what do we do if we suspect an auditory processing problem in a stuttering child? For example, should left brain dominance for auditory stimulation be strengthened by more auditory stimulation through earphones to the right ear?

Starkweather's monograph, *Stuttering and Laryngeal Behavior: A Review* (1982), and Hanley's paper at the conference reflect the renewed interest since about 1970 in minimal motor factors and stuttering. Wingate's studies of adults (Wingate, 1976) were probably the beginning of this development. In reaction time studies employing brief verbal responses (vowels or consonant-vowel combinations), the general conclusion is that stutterers show longer latencies. Some evidence for a more general or overall minimal motor difference is Luper and Cross' (1978) finding that stutterers (5 year olds, 9 year olds, and adults) differ from matched non-stutterers on both a voice reaction time task and a finger reaction time response. The correlations of scores on the two types of tasks were very high: + .96 for the stutterers and + .88 for the non-stutterers. It should be noted that Reich, Till and Goldsmith (1981), in a study similar to Luper and Cross', but using adult subjects only, found a difference between stutterers and non-stutterers on speech reaction time, but not for forefinger button pressing or a throat clearing cough. They concluded that the longer speech reaction times exhibited by the stutterers "reflect learned anticipatory fears of phonatory initiation and maladaptive prephonatory muscular sets." (p. 195). In other words, emotional conditioning could be involved in the minimal motor reaction time differences found. The problem of separating out these factors, i.e., a motor response difference as being due to neurophysiological factors or minimal emotional factors, seems to be a very formidable one.

Hanley stresses that studies of motor processes in children who stutter must focus on various levels of the speech production system (neural, muscular, emotional, etc.) simultaneously, and moreover, the interaction of the child and the environment must be considered in doing meaningful research and clinical study. We appreciate Hanley's understanding of the complexity

---

*For a review of information on auditory processes in stutterers, see Gregory and Mangan (1982).

of the tasks before us. Nevertheless, studies of motor and linguistic factors have perhaps directed us to a consideration of these child developmental characteristics as possible contributing factors in a child beginning to stutter. For many years (Gregory, 1968, 1973b, 1979) I have speculated on what I have considered to be an almost embarrassing simplification: that the physiological differences in beginning stuttering children that contribute to an increase of irregular syllable repetitions or prolongations in their speech are very minimal ones and probably vary from child to child with reference to the way that cognitive-linguistic-motor functioning is affected. If these factors were of a greater magnitude there would be a more apparent expressive speech production problem.

Communicative stress and interpersonal stress are viewed by all clinicians and researchers as important in the development and maintenance of stuttering. As mentioned earlier, those who have examined the possibility of genetic factors assume that environmental conditions interact with genetic predispositions (Kidd, 1977). Based on parental interviews and observations of parents interacting with the child while communicating, we have observed communicative stress factors (for example, parents who talk rapidly and seem to almost never pause) and interpersonal stress factors (for example, parent-parent conflict or parent-child conflict).

In his presentation concerned with emotional and environmental factors, Williams emphasizes looking at the beginning of stuttering in a child as a *communication problem* involving, (1) Stress children impose upon themselves, e.g., attempting vocabulary and sentences that are beyond their maturation-learned abilities, (2) Stress imposed by the listener, e.g., being impatient with the child as he talks or interrupting, and (3) Stress stemming from ambivalent feelings, e.g., when there are feared consequences for what is being said or when the parents expect perfectionism not only in their child, but also in themselves.

While there has been a great deal of research relating to personality characteristics of parents of stuttering children and the children themselves, the procedures available for this type of research have been of questionable validity. In my opinion, a particularly useful approach during the last 15 years has been the investigation of parent-child interactive behavior in a more objective manner. Kasprisn (1970) and Kasprisn-Burrelli, Egolf, and Shames (1972) trained observers to reliably identify parents' positive and negative child directed behaviors. Observation indicated that parents of stuttering children exhibited more negative verbal profiles than parents of non-stuttering children. They also reported that the negative profiles of parents talking to stuttering children became less negative following treatment in which the parents participated. Mordecai (1979) conducted a study in which parent-child triads (mother, father, child) were videotaped during a prescribed activity period designed to provide opportunities for parents to instruct, compete, converse, and play with their pre-school children. Parents of children beginning to stutter were found to allow inadequate opportunities for their child to respond to questions before asking another question or making another statement. Parents of non-stuttering children were found to comment more frequently upon the content of their child's preceding utterance, this being generally regarded as a positive behavior.

Gregory and Hill (1980) have observed the following interactive behaviors as important in the development and maintenance of stuttering: interruption, filling in words, finishing the child's statement, guessing what the child is about to say, asking multiple questions at once, constant correction of the child's verbal and nonverbal behavior, and speech models of rapidly paced conversation including quickly changing topics.

Although the interaction analysis is more objective, environmental factors contributing to increased disfluency may be recognized through the taking of a case history that includes a discussion of communication and interpersonal variables. A parent may have too high a level of expectation related to speech development or to behavior in general such as table manners and neatness. For many years, Sheehan (1970, 1975) has recommended considering how much support the child is receiving relative to how much is demanded, what he terms the demand/support ratio. Other factors, such as hectic or inconsistent family routine and crisis within the family (Wyatt, 1969) can be discovered through an interview.

Differential Evaluation — Differential Treatment

Based upon the presentations at the conference, as well as their own knowledge and experience, participants appeared to be in general agreement that clinicians are focusing on factors during evaluation and intervention aimed toward the prevention of stuttering, stemming the tide of beginning stuttering, or improving the fluency of a child with a more confirmed stuttering problem:

(1) Communicative stress in the environment, e.g., the way in which the parents talk to the child or the rates of the parents' speech.
(2) Interpersonal stress, e.g., the general interaction between family members.
(3) Linguistic and motoric developmental differences.
(4) Speech fluency.

It is assumed that the first three of these influence the fourth, but consideration is also given to using procedures that help the young child modify speech flow. Multiple etiology theories of VanRiper (1973) and others have always implied the necessity of a broad evaluation and several clinical writers (Gregory, 1973b; Riley and Riley, 1979; Gregory and Hill, 1980; Riley and Riley, 1983) have described differential therapy as based on differential evaluation. Of course, evaluation is a process that begins before treatment but certainly evaluation continues during therapy.

There is wide agreement that commonalities exist in intervention, but procedures have to be specific to some extent for each child. During the conference, all of the main speakers, regardless of whether they focused on emotional and environmental factors, linguistic, or motoric factors, described evaluation and treatment procedures that included the four components listed above. Everyone realizes the care that must be taken in making intervention decisions. The clinician may identify a principal contributing factor, but ordinarily several factors related to the child's development and environment are focused upon during successful intervention.

In many clinics, psychological consultation is routine and in others, referrals are made as the need is recognized. Oftentimes, clinical psychologists, social workers, or school counselors can be of assistance in our study of the child's environment (parental adjustment, parental attitudes, etc.) or in understanding subtle attitudes in stuttering children that the speech-language pathologist may not perceive. Information on perceptual and intellectual functioning that will relate to our study of speech and language processes can be provided by a clinical psychologist. A psychiatrist who attended the conference urged that speech-language pathologists explore relating more often to professionals in his field. He said, "Give us the chance to help." During the conference, whenever multidisciplinary cooperation was discussed, there was general agreement that multidisciplinary approaches should be used in evaluation and, when needed, in treatment. Clinicians should seek out professional resources in psychology, education, and medicine.

Prevention and Early Intervention Strategies

Much progress has been made in the generation of effective strategies for working with pre-school children showing various degrees of stuttering. Hanley, Nelson, and Williams describe their approaches in this book. Other participants in the conference have described their work with pre-school children elsewhere (Luper and Mulder, 1964; Adams, 1980; Costello, 1980, 1983; Gregory and Hill, 1980; Shine, 1980; Starkweather, 1980; Bailey and Bailey, 1982; Conture, 1982; Riley and Riley, 1983; Rustin, 1983).

When it has been decided that a child is disfluent, environmental manipulation is usually the first approach. Based on the observation of parent-child interaction and reports of the parents, recommendations are made for modifying the way in which the parents and others in the environment communicate with the child. Nelson provides excellent guidelines for this activity relating to the speech rate of the child and those around him, the way in which questions are asked, listening and attending, etc. For example, she points out that questions put children on the spot for a response and recommends reducing the number of questions asked by approximately 50%. Williams discusses reducing communicative stress, but he also makes suggestions for counseling the parents about more general environmental factors such as daily routines, disciplinary practices, and expectations for the child.

There seems to be general agreement that the effectiveness of environmental modification should be evaluated before it is decided to use more direct precedures, even modeling of easy-relaxed speech by the clinician, to improve the child's fluency. Gregory and Hill (1980) point out, however, that it may be necessary for the clinician to model changes in parent-child interaction for the parents and then reinforce the parents as they change their behavior during interactions with the child at the clinic. In our experience, this has been a successful approach.

Giving consideration to several factors, the clinician determines the nature of therapy for the child. The first factor is obviously what we have just mentioned, the child's responses to environmental changes. The second factor is the severity of the fluency difference or stuttering and the third is the length of time the problem has existed. The presence or absence of complicating speech, language, or behavioral problems is a fourth consideration. If stuttering is more severe or has been present for six months or longer, environmental manipulation may not be as successful, and focusing on the modification of speech flow may be necessary. Complicating problems of speech or behavior usually require clinical attention. Nelson states that three behaviors signal a need for direct intervention to modify speech flow: (1) breath stream mismanagement and/or hard vocal attacks, (2) active attempts to stop stuttering, and (3) active attempts to conceal stuttering. She provides a detailed description of her approach.

We noted during the conference that Cooper (1976, 1979) has described the use of fluency enhancing gestures and that Gregory (1973a), VanRiper (1973), Perkins (1979), Gregory and Hill (1980), and Shine (1980) have described the modeling by the clinicians of modifications in the child's speech that result in normal fluency by focusing on the minimal number of parameters necessary. For one child a slower rate with easy initiations may be all that is required. Another child may, for example, require attention to the reduction of vocal tension beginning with isolated vowels and a breathy approach.

An issue usually discussed when considering fluency problems in children, is the problem of working with the child who also manifests a language or articulation problem, or both. Clinicians appear to have resolved this matter during recent years. Procedures to facilitate fluency are usually carried out in the context of a language activity program working from shorter to longer utterances and from less meaningful to more meaningful content. Therefore, language therapy can be integrated with procedures to facilitate fluency. In addition, as the child is responding positively and fluency is improving, articulation can be focused upon using a relaxed, developmental approach. Clinicians who know language and articulation therapy, as well as stuttering therapy, will recognize how all of these activities can be integrated.

Therapy for Children with More Confirmed Stuttering Problems

In general, I refer here to school aged children. Each year of maturity is an important variable in therapy. What the child can understand will depend on cognitive development and more active cooperation will relate to interest and motivation. Just as was true with pre-school children, communicative stress and interpersonal stress are important factors to be managed by the clinician. What has been said about articulation and language problems in discussing pre-school children applies here taking age into consideration. Clinicians agree widely that procedures should be used with the school aged group to enhance the child's confidence in his ability to speak easily and enjoy communication. Analysis of stuttering behavior may be counterproductive. Williams (1979) emphasizes focusing on the overall way of talking. Nelson's fluency building strategies are appropriate. I have found considerable success in using a less specific approach at first in which the clinician models "more easy relaxed speech with smooth movements" beginning with short utterances and working up to longer and more complex ones in more propositional situations. More specific analysis of the child's speech and work on modification is used only to the extent necessary.

For therapy to be effective, it should be fairly intensive at first, i.e., at least three individual sessions of 30-50 minutes a week. One of the problems of effective stuttering therapy in the public schools has been the infrequency and short duration of therapy sessions. Another difficulty has been inadequate counseling with parents.

In a very recent publication, Thompson (1983) has described a program of differential therapy for school aged children and offered some of the best comment available on working with children in the school setting. During the conference, Thompson urged participants, through school and community educational programs, to become stronger advocates of the needs of the child who stutters.

Transfer and Maintenance

At all ages, transfer and maintenance is a crucial aspect of change. Stimulus generalization enhances transfer, but clinicians also plan activities in which responses made successfully in one situation are practiced in another. Maintenance of change over time is related to the effectiveness of therapy in general, but clinicians also plan specific activities aimed toward the retention of therapeutic effects. We have referred earlier in this chapter to the clinician modeling changes in interactive behaviors for the parents. We have also discussed the way in which the clinician models change in speech for the child and for the parents.

Gradually, the parents take part in therapy, participating for short and then longer periods. In the normal progression, parents are given assignments to do at home just what they have done at the clinic. In this way, the parents and the child are experiencing generalization and transfer. Maintenance usually consists of telephone checks with the parents and rechecks of the child at six month intervals at the clinic or in the home. We must stay in touch with the parents until we are satisfied that speech is developing normally.

Increased planning for effective transfer of change and the clinician's accepting responsibility for maintenance has been a major development in stuttering therapy during the last decade. Better planning of generalization and transfer and follow-up for 18-24 months following a period of treatment is a challenge for the future.

Measurement Procedures

Clinicians can identify stuttering behaviors reliably and thus count the percentage of syllables or words stuttered. Ordinarily, within word breaks in fluency, one syllable word repetitions, and accessory or struggle behaviors (sometimes referred to as secondary behaviors) are defined as stuttered. The clinician keeps in mind what we have said about most children showing infrequent syllable repetitions and prolongations and considerable repetition of one syllable words.

More and more clinicians are counting disfluencies, including borderline atypical ones and more atypical or stuttered behaviors during evaluation. Furthermore, progress is being charted in terms of speech measures such as percentage of syllables or words stuttered and rate in syllables or words per minute.

The validity of measures of change in speech to the natural environment continues to be a problem. The practicing clinician should realize that there are differences between overt measures (the subject knowing that a recording is being made) and covert measures (the subject not knowing that a recording is being made). However, this difference is probably minimal for preschool children.

Ingham is well known for the attention he has given to the problem of making valid assessments of stuttering behavior, considering the variability of disfluency in children and stuttering behavior itself. His chapter focuses on a recommended time series of assessments before, during, and following therapy. He provides rationale for within and beyond-clinic recorded assess-

144

ments twice weekly over at least four weeks before therapy, the same frequency during therapy including the transfer phase and finally, the same frequency for at least four weeks during maintenance. Conference participants were very interested in Ingham's method of integrating maintenance and outcome evaluation strategies by extending the length of time between follow-up assessments if the subject maintains prescribed criteria when evaluated. In this way the person is rewarded for successful maintenance of change. This is a strategy for older children and adults. With pre-school children, this may be motivating to the parents.

Quite obviously, we must make measures of the speech behavior that is our target in therapy as well as other variables we consider important, e.g., parent-child interaction. The basic instrument needed is a good tape recorder. Ingham understands the time limitation problems of practicing clinicians, but he urges refinement of measures to make therapy more effective, and I may add, to make clinical evaluation and treatment more interesting for the clinician.

The Future

There appears to be reason for considerable optimism about progress being made in the evaluation of children's fluency, identification of factors contributing to the development and maintenance of stuttering, and the making of decisions about intervention. Clinicians, such as those attending the Evanston conference, need to describe their work more carefully through case study reports including data on fluency and other variables. More clinicians should take steps to improve their skills, or become specialists in the treatment of stuttering, by going to centers where effective work is underway for observation and instruction. School programs, hospitals, and universities should sponsor more workshops and other continuing education opportunities in which information like that in this book can be shared and discussed. Children and parents should be referred to clinicians who have proven competence in the area of stuttering therapy, or ones who are working under the supervision of an experienced person.

Basic research about the nature of fluency, disfluency, and stuttering should continue and this information should be made available to practicing clinicians as we have done in this book and at the conference in 1982.

References

Adams, M., "A Clinical Strategy for Differentiating the Normally Nonfluent Child and the Incipient Stutterer," *Journal of Fluency Disorders*, 2, 141-149, 1977.

Adams, M., "The Young Stutterer: Diagnosis, Treatment, and Assessment of Progress," in Perkins, W. (Ed.), *Strategies in Stuttering Therapy*. New York: Thieme-Stratton, 1980.

Bailey, A., and Bailey, W., "Managing the Environment of the Stutterer," in Luper, H. (Ed.), "Intervention With the Young Stutterer," *Journal of Childhood Communication Disorders*, 6, 1982.

Blood, G., and Seider, R., "The Concomitant Problems of Young Stutterers," *Journal of Speech and Hearing Disorders*, 46, 31-33, 1981.

Brownell, W., *The Relationship of Sex, Social Class, and Verbal Planning to the Disfluencies Produced by Non-stuttering Pre-school Children*. Unpublished doctoral dissertation, Buffalo, State University of New York, 1973.

Conture, E., *Stuttering*. Englewood Cliffs, New Jersey: Prentice-Hall, 1982.

Cooper, E. B., "The Development of a Stuttering Chronicity Prediction Checklist for School Aged Stutterers: A Research Inventory for Clinicians," *Journal of Speech and Hearing Research*, 38, 215-223, 1973.

Cooper, E. B., *Personalized Fluency Control Therapy: An Integrated Behavior and Relationship Therapy for Stutterers*. Austin, Texas: Learning Concepts, 1976.

Cooper, E. B., "Intervention Procedures for the Young Stutterer," in Gregory, H. (Ed.), *Controversies About Stuttering Therapy*. Baltimore: University Park Press, 1979.

Costello, J., "Operant Conditioning and the Treatment of Stuttering," in Perkins, W. (Ed.), *Strategies in Stuttering Therapy*. New York: Thieme-Stratton, 1980.

Costello, J., "Current Behavioral Treatments for Children," in Prins, D., and Ingham, R. (Eds.), *Treatment of Stuttering in Early Childhood: Methods and Issues*. San Diego: College-Hill Press, 1983.

Curlee, R., "A Case Selection Strategy for Young Disfluent Children," in Perkins, W. (Ed.), *Strategies in Stuttering Therapy*. New York: Thieme-Stratton, 1980.

Curry, F. K. W., and Gregory, H. H., "The Performance of Stutterers on Dichotic Listening Tasks Thought to Reflect Cerebral Dominance," *Journal of Speech and Hearing Research*, 12, 73-82, 1969.

DeJoy, D., *An Investigation of the Frequency of Nine Individual Types of Disfluency and Total Disfluency in Relation to Age and Syntactic Maturity in Non-stuttering Males, Three and One Half Years of Age and Five Years of Age*. Unpublished doctoral dissertation, 155-158, Evanston, Illinois, Northwestern University, 1975.

Gregory, H., "Modeling Procedure in the Treatment of Elementary School Age Children Who Stutter," *Journal of Fluency Disorders*, 1, 58-63, 1973a.

Gregory, H., *Stuttering: Differential Evaluation and Therapy*. Indianapolis: Bobs-Merrill, 1973b.

Gregory, H., and Hill, D., "Stuttering Therapy for Children," in Perkins, W. (Ed.), *Strategies in Stuttering Therapy*. New York: Thieme-Stratton, 1980.

Gregory, H., and Mangan, J., "Auditory Processes in Stutterers," in Lass, N. (Ed.), *Speech and Language: Advances in Basic Research and Practice.* New York: Academic Press, 1982.

Hall, J. W., and Jerger, J. "Central Auditory Function in Stutterers," *Journal of Speech and Hearing Research*, 21, 324-337, 1978.

Hall, P., "The Occurrence of Disfluencies in Language-disordered School-age Children," *Journal of Speech and Hearing Disorders*, 42, 364-369, 1977.

Haynes, W., and Hood, S., "Disfluency Changes in Children as a Function of the Systematic Modification of Linguistic Complexity," *Journal of Communicative Disorders*, 11, 79-93, 1977.

Johnson, W., *Stuttering in Children and Adults.* Minneapolis: University of Minnesota Press, 1955.

Kasprisn, A., *Implications of Parental Verbal Behavior for Stuttering Therapy with Children.* Unpublished paper, American Speech and Hearing Association Convention, New York, 1970.

Kasprisn-Burrelli, A., Egolf, D., and Shames, G., "A Comparison of Parental Verbal Behavior with Stuttering and Non-stuttering Children," *Journal of Communication Disorders*, 5, 335-346, 1972.

Kidd, K. K., "A Genetic Perspective on Stuttering," *Journal of Fluency Disorders*, 2, 259-269, 1977.

Kowal, S., O'Connell, D. C., and Sabin, E. F., "Development of Temporal Patterning and Vocal Hesitations in Spontaneous Narratives," *Journal of Psycholinguistics Research*, 4, 195-207, 1975.

Luper, H. L., and Mulder, R., *Stuttering: Therapy for Children.* Englewood Cliffs, New Jersey: Prentice-Hall, 1964.

Luper, H. L., and Cross, D. E., *Finger Reaction Time of Stuttering and Non-stuttering Children and Adults.* Paper presented at the Annual Convention of the American Speech and Hearing Association, San Francisco, 1978.

Merits-Patterson, R., and Reed, C., "Disfluencies in the Speech of Language-Disordered Children," *Journal of Speech and Hearing Research*, 24, 55-58, 1981.

Mordecai, D., *An Investigation of the Communicative Styles of Mothers and Fathers of Stuttering Versus Non-stuttering Pre-school Children During a Triadic Interaction.* Unpublished doctoral dissertation, 48-64, Evanston, Illinois, Northwestern University, 1979.

Perkins, W., "From Psychoanalysis to Discoordination," in Gregory, H. (Ed.), *Controversies About Stuttering Therapy.* Baltimore: University Park Press, 1979.

Quinn, P. T., "Stuttering, Cerebral Dominance and the Dichotic Word Test," *Medical Journal of Australia*, 2, 639-643, 1972.

Reich, A., Till, J., and Goldsmith, H., "Laryngeal and Manual Reaction Times of Stuttering and Non-stuttering Adults," *Journal of Speech and Hearing Research*, 24, 192-196, 1981.

Riley, G., and Riley, J., "A Component Model for Diagnosing and Treating Children Who Stutter," *Journal of Fluency Disorders*, 4, 279-294, 1979.

Riely, G., and Riley, J., "Evaluation as a Basis for Intervention," in Prins, D., and Ingham, R. (Eds.), *Treatment of Stuttering in Early Childhood: Methods and Issues.* San Diego: College-Hill Press, 1983.

Rustin, L., "Intervention Procedures for the Disfluent Child," in Dalton, P. (Ed.), *Approaches to the Treatment of Stuttering.* Beckenham, Kent (England): 1983.

St. Louis, K., "Linguistic and Motor Aspects of Stuttering," in Lass, N. (Ed.), *Speech and Language: Advances in Basic Research and Practice.* New York: Academic Press, 1978.

Sheehan, J. (Ed.), *Stuttering: Research and Therapy.* New York: Harper and Row, 1970.

Sheehan, J., "Conflict Theory and Avoidance-reduction Therapy," in Eisenson, J. (Ed.), *Stuttering: A Second Symposium.* New York: Harper and Row, 1975.

Shine, R., "Direct Management for the Beginning Stutterer," in Perkins, W. (Ed.), *Strategies in Stuttering Therapy.* New York: Thieme-Stratton, 1980.

Sommers, R., Brady, W., and Moore, W. H., "Dichotic Ear Preference of Stuttering Children and Adults," *Perceptual and Motor Skills,* 41, 931-938, 1975.

Starkweather, W., "A Multiprocess Behavioral Approach to Stuttering Therapy," in Perkins, W. (Ed.), *Strategies in Stuttering Therapy.* New York: Thieme-Stratton, 1980.

Starkweather, W., "Stuttering and Laryngeal Behavior: A Review," *ASHA Monographs,* 21, 1982.

Thompson, J., *Assessment of Fluency in School-age Children.* Danville, Illinois: Interstate, 1983.

Toscher, M. M., and Rupp, R. R., "A Study of the Central Auditory Processes in Stutterers Using the Synthetic Sentence Identification (SSI) Test Battery," *Journal of Speech and Hearing Research,* 21, 779-792, 1978.

VanRiper, C., *The Treatment of Stuttering.* Englewood Cliffs, New Jersey: Prentice-Hall, 1973.

VanRiper, C., *The Nature of Stuttering.* Englewood Cliffs, New Jersey: Prentice-Hall, 1982.

Wexler, K., and Mysak, E., "Disfluency Characteristics of 2-, 4-, and 6-year-old Males," *Journal of Fluency Disorders,* 7, 37-46, 1982.

Wingate, M. E., *Stuttering: Theory and Treatment.* New York: Irvington, 1976.

Wyatt, G., *Language Learning and Communication Disorders in Children.* New York: The Free Press, 1969.

Yairi, E., "Disfluencies of Normally Speaking Two-year-old Children," *Journal of Speech and Hearing Research,* 24, 490-495, 1981.

Yairi, E., "Longitudinal Studies of Disfluencies in Two-year-old Children," *Journal of Speech and Hearing Research,* 25, 155-160, 1982.